Managing your Multiple Sclerosis

Comments on *Managing your Multiple Sclerosis*

'The book is well written, clear and accurate – it will be a good reference book for people with MS.'

DR SANDY BURNFIELD, Stockbridge

Managing your Multiple Sclerosis

Practical advice to help you manage your multiple sclerosis

Ian Robinson MA

*Director of the Brunel MS Research Unit,
Department of Human Sciences,
Brunel University, West London*

and

Dr F Clifford Rose FRCP

Director of the London Neurological Centre

CLASS PUBLISHING · LONDON

Printing history
First published 2004

The authors and publishers welcome feedback from the users of this book. Please contact the publishers.

Class Publishing, Barb House, Barb Mews, London, W6 7PA, UK
Telephone: 020 7371 2119 [International +4420]
Fax: 020 7371 2878
Email: post@class.co.uk
Visit our website – www.class.co.uk

The information presented in this book is accurate and current to the best of the authors' knowledge. The authors and publisher, however, make no guarantee as to, and assume no responsibility for, the correctness, sufficiency or completeness of such information or recommendation. The reader is advised to consult a doctor regarding all aspects of individual health care.

A CIP catalogue record for this book is available from the British Library

ISBN 1 85959 071 3

Edited by Michèle Clarke

Designed and typeset by Martin Bristow

Illustrations by David Woodroffe

Indexed by Val Elliston

Printed and bound in Finland by WS Bookwell, Juva

Contents

Note to reader

Managing Your Multiple Sclerosis is not a book about what MS is, its causes and diagnosis. It is a practical guide to its management and there is more information to be found in *Multiple Sclerosis – the 'at your fingertips' guide*, which can be found in your local bookshop, library or possibly your nearest health clinic; also the MS Society (details in Appendix 1) can provide you with many information sheets on this subject. This new book was written by popular demand from readers of the first book who wanted to know more about practical steps that they could take in their day-to-day living with MS.

There is a glossary at the end of this book to help you with any words that may be unfamiliar to you. If you are looking for particular topics, you can use either the detailed list of Contents on pp. v–viii or the Index, which starts on p. 234.

1
Multiple sclerosis explained

Managing Your Multiple Sclerosis is not a book about what MS is, its causes and diagnosis. It is a practical guide to its management and there is more information than is given in this introductory chapter to be found in *Multiple Sclerosis – the 'at your fingertips' guide*, which can be found in your local bookshop, library or possibly your nearest health clinic; also the MS Society (details in Appendix 1) can provide you with many information sheets on this subject. This new book was written by popular demand from readers of the first book who wanted to know more about practical steps that they could take in their day-to-day living with MS.

What is MS?

Damage to your nerves

MS is a disease of the central nervous system (CNS); it damages the protective coating around the nerve fibres (Figure 1.1) which transmit messages to all parts of your body, especially those controlling muscular and sensory activity. It is thought to be an 'autoimmune disease': this is where your body's own immune system appears to attack itself. As the damage to the protective coating around the nerve fibres – called 'myelin' – increases, it leads to a process known as 'demyelination' (Figure 1.2), where the coating is gradually destroyed. These nerves then become less and less efficient at transmitting messages. The messages, as it were, 'leak' from the nerve fibres where demyelination has occurred, rather like the loss of an electric current through a cable that is not insulated. As the messages 'leak', they become weaker and more erratic, thus leading to greater and greater difficulty in controlling muscles or certain sensory activities in various parts of your body.

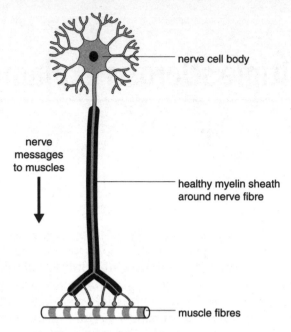

Figure 1.1 Healthy nerves.

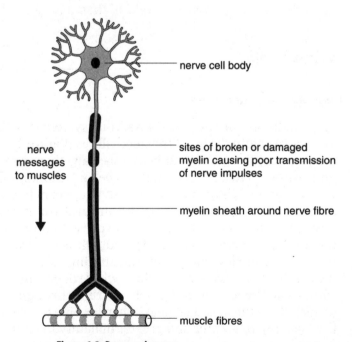

Figure 1.2 Damaged nerves

Problems of repair

Which nerve fibres are demyelinated, in which order, and at what rate, varies very widely between individuals, so the corresponding loss of muscular and sensory control also varies widely. Moreover, even when damage does occur to the myelin, it is sometimes gradually repaired (i.e. some remyelination occurs) through internal body repair mechanisms; also, what might be described as 'inflammation' at the site of the damage often becomes less over time. However, in MS the rate of repair is slower than the rate at which the myelin is damaged; so the damage tends to accumulate more and more throughout the CNS. This damage results in plaques or lesions, which take the form of patchy scarring (areas of multiple 'sclerosis') where the demyelination has occurred. Thus the name 'multiple sclerosis' has evolved.

Types of MS

There are almost as many different forms of MS as there are people with the disease. Each person with MS has a slightly different clinical (and symptom) profile; the precise course that any one person's MS will take is not as predictable with the kind of detail that many people with the condition – as well as their doctors – may wish for. In this context, scientists and doctors are always trying to refine their classification of types of MS, as they get to know more and more about the condition and its symptoms. You may therefore come across several slightly different ways of describing types of MS.

There are several main types usually described:

- **Relapsing-remitting MS.** Many cases initially take the form of what is generally described as relapsing-remitting MS. especially in younger people. Symptoms worsen during an 'attack' or 'relapse' or 'flare-up', may be at their worst for several days or a little longer, and then gradually improve in the following weeks.
- **Chronic progressive (or primary progressive) MS.** This describes another pattern where symptoms gradually worsen after the first 'episode' or 'attack', with a continuing increase in disability; often this will involve deterioration in bodily movement (described as motor symptoms) of one kind or another, or sensory performance (especially eyesight).
- **Benign MS.** This is a term sometimes used to describe a course of MS in which symptoms are relatively minor, or progression is so

slow that it is almost clinically imperceptible, or there are very few attacks or relapses over long periods of time – usually 15 years following diagnosis. There is growing evidence that the course of MS is likely to be initially more benign, almost irrespective of initial symptoms, for those people with fewer lesions (plaques) detectable in the CNS with a scan, compared to those who have a larger number. Unfortunately, the evidence from long-term research is that most benign 'cases' of MS do eventually result in significant symptoms and disability, even though this may not occur for 20 or 30 years after diagnosis.

- **Secondary progressive MS.** MS can also change its form so that, for example, relapsing-remitting MS may change into what is called secondary progressive MS – when a relatively steady decline begins to occur and remissions grow less frequent.

Finally, in case you hear this point from other sources (but don't worry about it unduly), there is what some think to be a very, very rare variant of MS (others think it might be a separate disease), that can lead to death in a few months. This is sometimes, although completely misleadingly, described as malignant MS. There are also other rare types (for example, opticospinal MS).

Symptoms of MS

There are many symptoms associated with MS that occur to a greater or lesser degree. Some are more debilitating than others; some cause more inconvenience. They can, for example, include problems with:

- urinary and bowel function
- pain and changes in sensation and dizziness
- tiredness
- depression and cognitive or memory impairment
- mobility
- speech and eating difficulties
- problems with eyesight and hearing.

'Attacks' and 'remissions'

Symptoms of MS often appear quite suddenly, although they may be relatively mild early in the disease, as the protective myelin sheath of the nerve concerned is damaged so much (see earlier section) that the transmission of messages to the muscles or sensory organs is interrupted. Sometimes this process affects one set of nerves, and sometimes it affects several sets. This is often called 'an episode', or 'attack' or, when it recurs, an 'exacerbation', 'relapse' or 'flare-up' of MS.

Symptoms may almost disappear as some repair of the myelin takes place, particularly early in the disease, and 'inflammation' or swelling around the damaged areas subsides over the course of a few hours or sometimes days. When such symptoms disappear or become less severe, this process is usually called 'a remission', but there is always likely to be some residual damage to the nerves involved. Thus the same symptom is likely to reappear again, but this may not be for days, weeks, months, and sometimes for many years. As the disease progresses, damage will occur at new nerve sites and, from time to time, new symptoms will appear.

Some people have one or two attacks or relapses and then there are no further symptoms for many years. At the other extreme some people may experience almost continuous progression without any distinct remissions or attacks, but just a general decline in either sensory or muscle control, or both. In between these two extremes is the most frequent pattern of MS, consisting of shorter periods of attacks or relapses, separated by longer periods of gradual recovery, i.e. remissions.

Progression of symptoms

MS is known as a *progressive neurological disease*, even though we are still not good at predicting when, how and in what ways it will progress. Most people will experience a recurrence of the same symptoms that they had before, although the degree and the timing of that recurrence is difficult to judge precisely.

From time to time, new symptoms will probably appear, as the course of the disease affects another nerve pathway. It is hard to say what those new symptoms will actually be in any individual. They may be linked in some way to those you have already experienced, but completely new *sensory* or *motor* (movement-related) *symptoms* may appear. It is important, however, not to be constantly preoccupied in waiting for a new symptom to appear. It may occur in weeks or months, but you may be one of the more fortunate people with MS who never has another new symptom.

As a very rough guide, at any one time about one-third of all people with MS appear to be experiencing no serious relapses, about one-third are having a distinct relapsing-remitting course with relapses of varying severity, and about one-third are experiencing a chronically progressive course. About one-third of all people with MS have serious disabilities and require significant everyday support, and a further third require what might be described as significant lifestyle adjustments to manage their lives with MS.

Symptoms that can catch you unawares

Two particular symptoms are reported by people with MS as having quite an effect on many aspects of everyday life in unexpected ways.

Fatigue

Lots of people with MS complain that they sometimes feel extra-ordinarily tired. This tiredness, which is usually described as MS fatigue, can be very unpredictable and difficult to manage. You need to pace yourself carefully and be prepared to adapt your life from day to day, even hour to hour. This fatigue and ways of managing it are discussed in Chapter 7.

Bladder problems

Up to 80–90% of people with MS have some problems of this kind, although the nature of these problems differs widely. Early on in the disease there may be very few difficulties: a little more 'urgency' perhaps, i.e. wanting to urinate more suddenly and possibly more often, or having some problems over control, e.g. unexpectedly leaking a little. Whilst these particular problems may be considered medically to be modest or minor, for people with MS they involve quite a lot of thought and careful planning. Much later in the disease process these problems can become substantial, and require several strategies to manage them (discussed in Chapter 4).

An important point concerning all bladder problems associated with MS is that some recent studies have found a high proportion of those with urinary problems also have bladder infections that may exacerbate those problems considerably, as well as possibly causing pain. Such infections can be cured, in most cases with appropriate antibiotic treatment. So get help from your doctor on this issue and don't just assume that all your difficulties with your bladder are caused directly by the MS itself.

Outlook

Medium term

In general the progression of MS is slowest, and the outlook (often called the *prognosis*), is best for people who are diagnosed under the age of 40, and who have an initial relapsing-remitting history. However, the long-term prognosis, even in these cases, is impossible to predict with any certainty. A rather more helpful – although not entirely accurate – prediction can be made after assessing your disease for 5 years or so, taking into account the number as well as the severity of relapses over this period, and comparing your symptoms now with those 5 years previously. The working basis of the '5-year rule', as it is sometimes referred to, is that what has happened to you in the first 5 years will be a reasonable guide to what is going to happen in the medium term. Even this rule cannot be considered by any means infallible. It is just a guide.

Longer term

From recent research only about a third of people with MS appear to be seriously disabled, to the extent of requiring major assistance (such as a wheelchair) for their mobility, within 15 years following their diagnosis.

Many people – certainly when they are first diagnosed, or indeed when they suspect they have MS – consider being in a wheelchair as the thing they most fear about the disease, and what they most wish to avoid (see the section on *Chairs and wheelchairs* in Chapter 8). This could be, in part, because of the premium our society places on being independent and mobile, and the ways in which people in wheelchairs have been treated in the past. Moreover, it is always difficult to picture yourself in the future, in a situation when you have less of something than you have now, but this will happen to all of us at some point, whether we have MS or not. The experience of life is that almost all of us adapt to such situations pretty well when they occur, even though in prospect they may be rather daunting. In any case, as far as both coping with mobility and the public perception of people in wheelchairs go, there is a positive change taking place.

Management of symptoms

Symptom management in MS is often a complicated process. The symptoms may occasionally be wide ranging and so variable that a variety of strategies are often required:

- lifestyle changes
- drug therapies
- psychological or counselling support
- physiotherapy, speech and occupational therapies
- use of equipment
- home modifications
- and, in some cases, surgery.

Many symptoms or disabilities involve using more than one of these strategies, depending on their seriousness. The most important approach for all those involved in managing your symptoms is to find an appropriate balance between all the strategies, especially when several symptoms occur at the same time. There is much more about managing the symptoms and lifestyle changes in the rest of this book.

The causes of MS

The cause or causes of MS are still unknown. Although there are significant geographical variations in the distribution of people with MS throughout the world, a great deal of research has failed to uncover any tangible evidence that there are specific avoidable risk factors associated with the onset of the disease.

Genetic versus environmental causes

At present, the most likely cause appears to be a combination of genetic and environmental factors. Studies of identical twins, where one or both has MS, offer what might be called the 'purest' way in which to investigate this theory: it appears that genetic factors contribute between 30 and 35% and environmental factors about 65–70% of the total contribution to the cause. These two figures suggest that further research needs to be undertaken on both issues. There does not seem to be one simple gene linked to MS, but we do know, for example, that first-degree blood relatives of someone with MS, such as children and siblings (brothers and sisters), are at slightly enhanced risk of the disease.

Amongst many other theories about the causes of MS, there has been a particular interest in the role of 'heavy metals'. It is certainly true that an excess of some heavy metals in the body, such as lead, mercury and cadmium, may result in serious neurological damage. *Lead* in particular is a potential cause of neurological damage, although, with the reduction of lead in petrol, it is gradually being reduced in our environment, but at present there is no evidence that excess lead causes MS. Excess *mercury* can also produce neurological damage, and there has been much discussion about the possible problems with mercury-based dental fillings. However, a large proportion of the adult population will have had at least some mercury fillings in their lifetimes, and yet only a fraction of those people have MS. Dental amalgam does contain mercury which can erode over time and be absorbed into the bloodstream, but this is a very small contribution to the amount of mercury ingested by most people (deep-sea fish is a much greater source). The exposure to dental amalgam is well within the safety limits currently recommended for mercury.

Infections and other diseases

Research has not shown MS to be caused by any particular bacterial or viral infection, but it is possible that the timing of a relapse may coincide with an infection. This could be due to a change in immune activity that allows the infection to gain hold: the bacterial infection can trigger an immune response, or both the relapse and the infection may occur in response to some unknown third factor.

Candida

At present there is a widespread interest, particularly amongst many involved in alternative or complementary medicine, in *Candida albicans* (thrush). Although candida can be associated with many symptoms, as well as having a low-level but debilitating effect on health, there is almost no formal evidence that it is associated with relapses of MS in itself. Candida infection may be a result rather than a cause of a weakened immune system, and it is also known to be more common as a side effect of some anti-inflammatory drugs used in MS. Of course, any infection with potentially problematic symptoms should be treated with antibiotics.

Herpes

Amongst viruses that have prompted scientific interest in relation to MS, the herpes virus HHV-6 is one of a number currently being researched. However, as with other viral candidates for a cause of MS, this line of enquiry is controversial and much debated.

Lyme disease

There is no evidence that this disease, which is spread by tics living on a range of animal species in the countryside, can cause MS, although its symptoms may mimic those of MS.

'Flu jabs and other injections

Many people with MS naturally look for a preceding event, such as a 'flu jab, to explain why their symptoms have worsened, or why they have had an 'attack' or 'relapse'. Research studies have failed to demonstrate any link between injections (vaccinations or inoculations) and any subsequent worsening of the MS.

Links between MS and other conditions including cancer

Many people with MS can point to symptoms and illnesses that seem to have preceded its onset. There is no clear definitive link that been established between the prior effects of diseases and the onset of MS. Of course as MS progresses, it may itself give rise, in effect, to other conditions, through a weakened immune system or just by ageing, for example.

There is no known link between cancer of any type and MS, but it is to be expected that some people with MS will develop cancer, but no more frequently than people who do not have MS.

Autoimmune diseases

There are strong similarities between some aspects of other autoimmune diseases, where the immune system is triggered into mistakenly attacking normal tissues in the body, and some aspects of MS. At present these conditions are still thought to be completely separate disease entities, although it is possible that there may be some very general biological processes underlying these conditions. These processes are the object of considerable recent research.

Stress

Fatigue, and possibly what we call 'stress', could have had some effect, not as a cause of MS, but perhaps as an exacerbating factor on some symptoms. However, although most people with MS probably feel that undue stress in their lives may bring on a relapse, scientifically this issue is still being argued over. Even so, many people have their own ideas about things that they feel are linked with their MS symptoms, and try to avoid them.

Accidents and injuries

Studies have compared accident and injury rates in people with MS who have had relapses and those who have not. Almost all have concluded that there is no significant difference in rates, or evidence to support trauma as causing or worsening MS. A more general issue is whether head injuries may have broken what is called the *blood–brain barrier* so that some parts of the CNS may themselves become contaminated and thus be damaged by the various blood products that are released. However, the relationship of any breach of the blood–brain barrier and the onset of MS is disputed.

Diet

There has also been extensive scientific research on MS and diet which may have some bearing in the medium and longer term on health in general.

There is substantial research indicating that what are called 'unsaturated fatty acids' – essential building blocks of the brain and nervous system – may be deficient in people with MS, which is why supplements containing these fatty acids have become popular. However, there is little evidence that taking supplements with the fatty acids has any major effect on MS. More generally, there is also little evidence that any particular diet has major effects on the course of MS, although some evidence suggests that a low-saturated fat diet may be beneficial as regards relapses.

Finally, there is little or no evidence that poor diet in itself causes MS – if this were so, the geographic and social distribution of MS would be very different.

Diagnosing MS

The diagnosis of MS has previously been a long, slow and complicated process, since there was no definitive laboratory test for MS. The newer and sophisticated brain scanning techniques that are now used, such as magnetic resonance imaging (MRI) can locate lesions or patchy scarring (scleroses) in the nervous system, but require very careful interpretation by a skilled doctor. Although many people in the early stages of MS do not exhibit the 'classic' symptoms considered to be the 'textbook' features of the disease, MRI can be the definitive test as it shows lesions in the white matter which contains myelinated fibres. Finally, many other conditions may produce symptoms almost indistinguishable from MS symptoms. Thus the difficulty in diagnosing MS lies in establishing sufficient evidence to exclude other possibilities. There is more about diagnosing MS in *Multiple Sclerosis – the 'at your fingertips' guide* (see Appendix 2).

2
Medical management of MS

Despite claims that are made from time to time, at present there is no scientifically validated cure for MS, neither can we prevent its onset, but we are now beginning to enter the era of what are becoming known as DMTs (disease-modifying therapies). In addition to the possibility of influencing the onset of attacks, lessening their effects and increasing the length of remissions, the possibilities of longer term disease modification are now being actively considered.

This chapter discusses the issues of treatment rather than cure, what medical therapies there are at present, and rehabilitation.

Treatment rather than cure

Repairing the damage

One of the reasons why MS is such a difficult disease to cure is that, once the CNS has been damaged, it would involve major repair of the often severe structural damage. Any further process of damage would have to be prevented as well as the previous structural damage being repaired. However, despite these difficulties, there is considerable interest in experimental work on drugs that may be able to 'remyelinate' damaged nerves, and drugs that may slow down or halt the process of further damage.

Symptom remission

Most claims for a cure for MS have been made on the basis that the symptoms seem to have disappeared, temporarily at least, but not that the structural damage of MS has been repaired. The problem is that symptoms of MS can be dormant for many years, or dramatic remissions in symptoms have occurred, but the damage to the CNS has not necessarily been repaired. Symptoms can reappear, and there is a significant possibility that they will do so, but without evidence that the underlying demyelination has been repaired, the disappearance of symptoms appears to be a temporary, although happy, coincidence; it is probably due to the absorption of fluid caused by the inflammatory response to demyelination. A number of newer drugs, particularly the beta-interferons and glatiramer acetate, may have some effects on modifying the disease process.

At present therefore, treatment mainly consists of:

- ameliorating a symptom or its effects;
- preventing or lessening the degree or length of time of a 'relapse';
- encouraging the early arrival of a 'remission';
- changing various aspects of your lifestyle that will make life with the symptoms of MS easier to manage;
- seeking to slow down the rate of progression of the disease.

In many cases, up until recently, the treatment of MS has been on the basis of symptoms as they occur. Now, in addition to attempts to reduce the number of relapses in MS, there are increasingly promising efforts to alter the course of MS itself. There are some drugs that offer the promise of lower rates of disease progression for some people, although for how many people and for how long is a subject of major controversy. Indeed the acronym DMT is now being used quite widely in discussions of MS, but we are still not talking about a cure, just a possibility of slower progression of the MS.

Approaches to treatment

There are now two basic approaches to treating MS medically.

First there are drugs that aim to suppress, minimize or halt the destructive immune response, that is the inflammation and the accompanying symptoms that occur when MS is in an active phase. In this context the overall aim is to move from controlling one or more relapses, to minimizing and ideally halting further disease progression. Steroid drugs have been used for many years to try and control the inflammation attending relapses and lessen symptoms, but they have little effect on the underlying disease. More recently, drugs based on beta-interferon and others based on glatiramer acetate are showing more promise in not only assisting in the control of relapses, but also appearing to modify the disease course in some people, as their effects seem to continue for several years. There are also as many as 50 promising individual therapies undergoing clinical trials at any one time, although few will end up being used in clinical practice, and the drugs are often targeted to only very specific types of the disease.

The second approach is to assess and treat the individual symptoms (e.g. spasticity, continence difficulties, pain or fatigue) that result from the damage to the CNS. In this respect there is no single drug treatment – an 'MS drug' – for all the symptoms of MS because of the immense variation and different rates of progression in each individual. Fortunately, MS is a condition where many symptoms can, in most cases, be relatively well managed for long periods of time.

The beta-interferons and the management of MS

What are beta-interferons?

Interferons are naturally occurring substances in the body, produced in response to 'invasion' by a foreign substance, such as a virus. Two different kinds of beta-interferons have shown a significant effect in MS by reducing the number and severity of its 'attacks': beta-interferon 1b (trade name Betaferon) and, more recently, beta-interferon 1a (trade names Avonex and Rebif). They seem to stabilize the immune system but there is conflicting evidence as to whether it also slows disease progression.

Who is helped by beta-interferons?

At present, this is not entirely clear. The drugs have been extensively tested on people with specific kinds of relapsing-remitting MS, mainly those in the earlier stages of MS and who can walk (in the jargon, those who were 'ambulant'). This was because it was easier to demonstrate the effectiveness of the drugs on people who were more mildly affected and who were having relatively regular 'relapses'. Findings of several trials showed that these people had a (statistically) significantly lower rate of relapses compared to a group of others who did not take the drugs and, furthermore, when they did have a relapse, it was likely to be less severe.

In the case of secondary progression, as it is preceded by a relapsing-remitting phase, such people may benefit through some of the therapies, which could have some effect on modifying the earlier phase of the disease.

In primary progressive MS, there is less compelling evidence at present that beta-interferons substantially affect the longer term course of the disease.

These current findings mean 'statistically' that there are still some people who took the drugs and who did not benefit a great deal from them. Beta-interferons may have less effect on people whose disease progression is substantial.

Nevertheless, at present, drug therapy for primary progressive MS is still mainly to manage any symptoms as they appear. However, given the evidence that beta-interferons can produce some benefits for both relapsing-remitting and secondary progressive MS, research is now increasingly interested in their potential effects in primary progressive MS.

Effects of beta-interferons

Expectations of the drugs have been so high that many people have been disappointed that they do not feel much better when they take them, but the drugs do not *cure* MS nor do they appear to repair existing damage: they just seem to slow down further damage and symptoms in some people, so both the original symptoms and any internal damage to your CNS will still be there. The drugs are working 'silently', thus, we anticipate, preventing some future symptoms and damage. You might wonder why you are taking drugs that you may think have no effect on your present symptoms!

The effect of beta-interferons, as far as we know, is to encourage the immune system to become more 'placid'. This seems to reduce the number and extent of the periodic 'inflammations' that lead to more MS symptoms; however, they do not necessarily *eliminate* those 'inflammations'. So relapses may still occur, even if they are fewer in number and less in degree than they would otherwise have been. The problem is that neither the doctor treating you, nor you yourself, know what would 'otherwise have been'. All you may know is that you now have (perhaps a minor) relapse, and are feeling worse. Your relapses might well have been worse without beta-interferon but, of course, you might feel that it was not effective at all.

Beta-interferons appear to work best when the disease is active, when (although not always) there are recognizable symptoms. The predominant medical opinion at present is that beta-interferons should be given only when there is evidence of recent disease activity, but the increasing research evidence that beta-interferons may slow down the development of symptoms over the medium term (3–5 years) is prompting a serious review of this position. Indeed, there are now scientifically influential voices arguing for the administration of beta-interferons at the earliest possible stage of the disease.

Longer term effects of beta-interferon

More studies will be needed to assess effects of beta-interferon over 15–20 years. We have data, at the time of writing this book, only on small groups of people who have had beta-interferons for 8–10 years, and this is not sufficient to make very long-term judgements. However, there are some promising signs. It does appear from current clinical trials that the onset or progression of disability, as measured by a range of tests, is slowed down by the beta-interferons and this slow-down is statistically significant – for at least 4 or 5 years after taking the drug. In addition, disease activity in the CNS as measured by magnetic resonance scans also seems to be reduced, but remember that most of these very positive results were obtained from people with milder forms of MS at an earlier stage of their disease.

A problem that has arisen in about a third of people being given beta-interferon 1b (Betaferon) is that they have developed 'antibodies' to the drug after about a year or so. It appears that their bodies are resisting the effects of beta-interferon, attacking beta-interferon as an 'invader'. In such cases, the positive effects of the drug disappear, and rate of relapses and disease progression returns – as far as we can see – to their previous state.

Another problem is that, at present, there is no test available to ascertain which people will develop these antibodies. It is mainly by the return of increased disease activity and symptoms that these people would recognize this problem. It is not clear whether exactly the same problems will occur with other types of beta-interferon, but the first signs are that they will.

How is beta-interferon given?

Beta-interferons may be currently administered in different ways. Beta-interferon 1b (Betaferon) is administered by injection subcutaneously (just below the skin) every other day. Beta-interferon 1a (Avonex) is administered by injection intramuscularly (directly into the muscles) every week. Beta-interferon 1a (Rebif) is administered subcutaneously three times a week. The different types of administration are based on what has proved in clinical trials to be the best way of ensuring the effectiveness of the drug.

Subcutaneous injections have been given in the past by a doctor or a nurse, not only to check that it is given correctly, but to monitor whether it is given at all – people are sometimes forgetful about administering any drug. However, this is a time-consuming and expensive method and some people now self-administer the drug, rather like insulin for people with diabetes. Intramuscular injections have to be given by a doctor (or nurse). Newer modes of administration are now being developed and trials are taking place to test whether these other methods are better and more effective.

None of the drugs can be taken by mouth (orally) as yet; they are proteins and likely to be broken down by the digestive processes, making them less effective, or possibly even ineffective.

How long is beta-interferon taken for?

Decisions will taken by your neurologist based on your personal situation, and taking into account:

- a longer term reduction in the number and degree of relapses compared to those you had before starting the beta-interferon;
- no substantial rise in unwanted side effects;
- no other clinical reason why you should not continue;
- no better therapies being available;
- the substantial financial issues involved, i.e. the cost of the drugs.

Side effects of beta-interferon

There have been two main side effects noted, mainly with beta-interferon 1b (Betaferon):

- There are symptoms best described as 'flu-like symptoms, which many, perhaps most, people experience in the first few months of treatment. These are generally mild and can be managed with ordinary analgesics (pain relievers), and they disappear in almost everyone after those first few months.
- Problems at the injection site, such as blotches or pain, which most people experience initially and about half some years later.

Such reactions are more of an irritation than anything else. Very rarely more serious reactions have been reported – only in a few cases serious enough to warrant stopping treatment.

As far as beta-interferon 1a drugs (Avonex and Rebif) are concerned, similar types of side effects were experienced, but at a lower rate.

We do not yet know about any longer term side effects, an important issue in MS where people usually live with their condition for several decades.

Controversies over the prescription of beta-interferon

As you may be aware, there has been great controversy over the availability of the expensive beta-interferons for people with MS on the NHS. An organization called NICE (the National Institute for Clinical Excellence) has been given responsibility by the UK government for the formal cost–benefit assessment of all drugs and medical devices. Only if NICE recommends that a drug or device is indeed sufficiently cost effective can it now be prescribed on the NHS, and even then there may be conditions about the circumstances in which it may be given or who may prescribe it. The issue for NICE, as far as the beta-interferons are concerned, has been what benefits occur, for what costs – remembering that the beta-interferons are very expensive drugs.

The assessment of beta-interferons was regarded as a priority for NICE because prescribing had already begun by certain neurologists in certain areas – leading to what was considered a 'postcode lottery' for people with MS. In fact in a Report issued in February 2002, NICE indicated that it did not believe that there was sufficient evidence at present to prescribe beta-interferons on the NHS. In other words their judgement was that prescription by the NHS was not currently cost effective. However, it indicated that people who had already been prescribed beta-interferons, before its judgement, could continue to receive them. It also indicated that efforts were being made to find ways for the drugs to be supplied on a more cost-effective basis.

In fact on the same day as the NICE announcement, it was also announced that what was called a 'risk-sharing agreement' had been reached with the relevant drug companies and the NHS to provide beta-interferons through neurologists in MS clinics for approximately 9000 people with MS (about 15% of those with the disease) on very specific criteria as follows:

Relapsing-remitting MS

People with MS must fulfil the following four criteria:

- be able to walk independently
- have had at least two clinically significant relapses in the last 2 years
- be 18 years old or older
- have no contraindications.

Secondary progressive MS

Beta-interferon is only prescribed for people with relapsing secondary progressive MS. It is not effective in people with a non-relapsing secondary progressive course. People must fulfil the following criteria:

- be able to walk at least 10 metres with or without assistance
- have had at least two disabling relapses in the last 2 years
- have had minimal increase in disability due to slow progression over the last 2 years
- be 18 years old or older

In relation to the agreement, a group of people with MS taking the drug will be evaluated over a period of 10 years, and the relationship of any benefits to the costs will be assessed. If the equation between costs and benefits is then considered as positive, the drugs will then be allowed to be prescribed on the NHS.

Compared to some other countries the proportion of those with MS being prescribed beta-interferons is still relatively low, although it should be said that, in addition to issue of cost, there is still substantial debate amongst neurologists as to the frequency and extent of benefits from the beta-interferons.

Glatiramer acetate (Copaxone) and the management of MS

Glatiramer acetate is a synthetic compound made of four amino acids (the building blocks of proteins) that are found in myelin. It has been shown in clinical trials that glatiramer acetate reduces the number and severity of relapses and appears to slow the onset of disability in some people with MS. While the mode of action of glatiramer acetate is not completely understood, it is different from that of the interferons.

Over the past 15 years, there have been many clinical trials to investigate the efficacy and safety of glatiramer acetate in people with MS. The best results were seen in people with MS who had the lowest levels of neurological disability. Studies have shown that at the end of 2 years there were about 25% fewer relapses in people taking glatiramer acetate compared with those not taking the drug, and more people on the drug tended to improve.

Administering glatiramer acetate

The drug is injected subcutaneously (under the skin) every day. People with MS or family members who first receive proper training in aseptic injection techniques can perform the injections without medical supervision.

Side effects of the drug

The drug is generally well tolerated and does not cause any of the 'flu-like symptoms or increase in depression sometimes associated with the interferon drugs. The most common side effects are injection site reactions, pain upon injection, and a postinjection reaction involving shortness of breath, flushing, palpitations, anxiety and chest pain. This reaction, which occurs in about one in seven people at one time or another resolves itself within 15–20 minutes and does not appear to have any long-term consequences. At the time it can, however, be very frightening.

Prescribing glatiramer acetate (Copaxone)

As the effect of glatiramer acetate and its process of development have been broadly similar to that of the interferons, it has also been subject to the same process of assessment by NICE as the interferons (see above). The same judgement was also made in relation to glatiramer acetate, as were also the same risk-sharing arrangements with the company manufacturing the drug. Thus the drug is also available for prescription by neurologists in MS clinics using slightly different criteria. To be prescribed the drug, people must fulfil the following criteria:

- be able to walk at least 100 metres without assistance
- have had at least two clinically significant relapses in the last 2 years
- be 18 years old or older.

The future of DMTs (disease-modifying therapies) in MS

It is undoubtedly true that we are in a very exciting phase of development of DMTs. Although we cannot yet talk about a cure, we can now consider seriously the possibility of slowing down the course of the disease and not just ameliorating the symptoms of relapses. However, the results of research so far seem to suggest that the earlier the current DMTs (the interferons and glatiramer acetate) are given in the course of the disease, the more effect they are likely to have. One current controversy is how early these drugs should be given. Some believe that they should be given at the very earliest sign of MS, others that these drugs should wait upon a full and clear diagnosis on more comprehensive criteria. Their cost is a major issue, particularly in relation to medium- and long-term benefits that have not yet been fully proven, and is a significant factor that has had to be considered by every healthcare system.

For people whose MS is more advanced, and particularly is progressive in nature, the effects of these DMTs seem to be very substantially less. As such people form the majority of those with MS at any one time, then many people will still feel disappointed that few possibilities exist for them in controlling their disease. However, there is very active research being undertaken at the moment to evaluate whether different combinations of any of the current DMTs could affect the course of MS for such people.

Steroids

Types

The use of steroid-based drugs for 'attacks' or 'relapses' of MS has been the standard treatment for MS for some years, and many people may still find that this is the first line of treatment offered to them.

There are several types of steroid drugs:

- **Adrenocorticosteroids** (such as ACTH – AdrenoCorticoTrophic Hormone), used to be one of the most commonly used steroids in MS.
- **Glucocorticosteroids** (such as prednisolone, given by mouth; or methylprednisolone, usually given through a drip, intravenously) are used more commonly now.

Effects of steroids

There is substantial evidence that both types reduce the inflammation at active disease sites in the CNS and, in particular, reverse disruptions of the blood–brain barrier (see Chapter 1) that may occur when the disease is active. These effects, in turn, should reduce the duration and degree of symptoms. However, most studies suggest that the effects of steroids are relatively short term, perhaps lasting a few weeks, although there have been one or two studies which suggest tantalizingly that there may be far longer positive effects of the combined short-term use of methyl-prednisolone and prednisolone.

There is also some interesting evidence from a trial on the use of steroids (methylprednisolone and prednisolone) following an initial episode of 'optic neuritis' (inflammation of the optic nerve, which makes things seem blurred). This is a significant symptom, which often acts as a forerunner of MS. There is more information on this trial in Chapter 18.

Overall there is a sense, at the moment, that further definitive trials to assess the most effective steroid, as well as its dose and mode of administration in MS, are now almost a waste of time and resources, as newer drugs – such as the beta-interferons, glatiramer acetate and others – show so much more promise for the control of MS, in relation not only to relapses, but also to the course of the disease.

How are steroids given?

ACTH has now been replaced by the use of methylprednisolone and prednisolone, but there is widespread debate amongst neurologists about the most appropriate steroid and mode of administration in MS. People with MS are likely to come across different ways in which steroids are currently given – intravenously administered methylprednisolone (called IVMP for short) normally requires a hospital stay for one to several days, depending on precisely how the drug is administered. There may need to be other hospital stays for assessment purposes.

Side effects

As with all powerful drugs, side effects – that is unwanted effects – can occur. Side effects appear to depend very much on both the type of steroid and how it is administered. When methylprednisolone is given in the usual short-term high intravenous doses, facial flushes, a metallic taste in the mouth during the treatment and sometimes acne occur. Most other reactions are not serious, but occasionally sleep disturbances, stomach upsets and mild mood changes occur. Very occasionally more serious psychological changes are seen.

With longer term administration of methylprednisolone, often followed by oral prednisolone, a range of unwanted effects may occur. These are very highly dependent on exactly how the steroids are given, for how long and the level of dose. Often signs of some water retention may occur: a 'moon-shaped face' and modest swelling (*oedema*) in several parts of the body. Normally, the cells of the body are bathed inside and outside in water, and this water is regulated by hormones, sodium (salt) levels and the kidneys. Steroids tend to cause the kidneys to retain sodium: an increase in sodium levels leads to an increase in water retention in the body, resulting usually in a modest but noticeable swelling – the oedema.

Steroids can also produce a temporary 'masculinization' in women through their hormonal effects, which can include increased body hair, menstrual irregularities, acne and, paradoxically, a loss of scalp hair. Very prolonged administration can produce a range of other effects, some of them very serious.

There is always a balance to be struck between probable improvement in some MS symptoms following a relapse, and the avoidance of as many of these side effects as possible. It may not be an easy decision for either the clinician or the person with MS. Usually the pressing nature of the symptoms produced by a relapse decides the immediate outcome. Nevertheless, the use of steroids must be very carefully monitored. The objective is to gain the maximum possible beneficial effects following dosage for the shortest possible time. However, longer term administration of steroids is thought on balance to be important in special circumstances, to try to contain the MS.

Getting more information on drug therapy

Side effects of drugs

Because drugs have powerful effects on a condition, they can also have powerful side (that is, unwanted) effects on other things. It is a good idea to be informed about the possible side effects of the drugs that you are taking; you will be able to assess the balance yourself between the effects and the side effects, and you will be alerted sufficiently to inform your GP, neurologist or MS Specialist Nurse about them, if they are worrying you.

Your medical practitioner (GP, neurologist or MS Specialist Nurse) should discuss possible side effects with you when your drug(s) are prescribed, including any side effects from combining two or more drugs. If your GP does not, you should ask explicitly about this issue. If you are still unclear or concerned, the pharmacist where you get your prescriptions has expert knowledge about drugs and their effects, and should be willing to answer questions about them. Furthermore, they can inform you about over-the-counter drug therapies that you may purchase, and their potential side effects and interactions with other drugs.

Several organizations (including the Consumers' Association and British Medical Association – see Appendix 1) publish excellent family health guides that contain detailed and up-to-date information about drugs and other treatments. It is vital that you use a British edition of any guide, as brand names are frequently changed from country to country. Some titles are included in Appendix 2 at the back of this book.

Combination therapy

Beta-interferon or glatiramer acetate and steroids can be taken at the same time but only after careful assessment by your neurologist. Even if you are taking beta-interferon 1b or beta-interferon 1a or glatiramer acetate, you may have a relapse, but probably to a lesser degree than you would have done without the treatment. In this situation, you may well be offered steroids – possibly a combination of methylprednisolone and prednisolone. The objective is to provide an additional means of reducing the inflammation, despite the use of beta-interferons, and reduce your symptoms.

Team approach to management

People with MS – and their relatives – often have questions and concerns about who is doing what when they go to see the various health practitioners.

It is relatively clear that your GP is medically responsible for your routine day-to-day health care. In the first instance you would normally go to your GP for advice about any symptoms, or other issues that concern you, even if they are not symptoms of MS. Most GPs will refer you on clinical grounds to support services for people with MS, often in the practice itself, such as nursing, counselling and, possibly, physiotherapy. Some larger general practices are also setting up multidisciplinary support clinics for patients with long-term conditions that, although not specifically targeted to MS, could be of value to people with the disease.

Once you have been referred to, and then been diagnosed by, a consultant (usually a neurologist), you would automatically become his or her patient as well in several ways:

- You will have hospital records with notes and records of your condition and, initially, you will be down as being under the care of the neurologist concerned.
- Most neurologists will want to assess you periodically – traditionally every 6 months – to evaluate how your MS is developing.
- Many neurologists are involved directly or indirectly in clinical

trials for new therapies for the disease or its symptoms, and they may invite you to participate in such trials, which will involve further regular monitoring or assessment (see Chapter 18).

- Particularly with the advent of beta-interferons and glatiramer acetate, possibly with certain other drugs, neurologists now have a special clinical role in dispensing them and monitoring their use.
- Both for clinical and economic reasons, hospitals are increasingly setting up MS clinics, and/or multidisciplinary support services for people with MS.

So, in principle, someone with MS could have an embarrassment of services, in both general practice and in a hospital setting! However, this is not usually the case. One of the major problems at present is that services are patchily distributed and relatively ill coordinated, and people with MS are having to take what is available to them. In the light of this unsatisfactory situation, the MS Society and leading neurologists have recently put together a minimum standard of service provision for people with MS, which they hope will lead to more consistent provision (see Appendix 2).

The situation is confused because, on the one hand, specialist advice and services in relation to your MS, i.e. those usually obtained through your neurologist and the hospital, take precedence over your GP's advice on the disease; on the other hand, your GP is responsible – as we noted earlier – for your day-to-day health care. The problem then becomes what is an MS-related problem, and what is not. Technically the GP and the specialist should be in touch with one another, informing each other of developments in relation to your health. This does not always happen efficiently.

The best advice to you is to use whichever local services are most convenient and helpful for whatever problems you happen to have, and to press your GP and/or the consultant as necessary for other services that you feel have not been offered. To be frank, what most people with MS have found is that their GP is helpful, supportive and accessible, but is often not particularly knowledgeable about MS, and that the consultant is knowledgeable but not as supportive or as accessible as the GP. The advent of MS clinics with other professional staff, such as nurses, as primary advisers may provide more support in due course.

The idea of a 'team approach' to MS has gained considerable ground in recent years and most neurologists and hospitals support it. In the previous ('non-team') approach, a doctor, usually the neurologist, might have referred you independently occasionally for separate professional services, e.g. physiotherapy, occupational therapy, speech therapy or nursing. People with MS often found this a problem in that each professional dealt with them independently; there seemed to be little communication between the different services, and no single person to whom they could turn for an overall view, apart from the neurologist who was not always accessible. You may be lucky in that you have access to an MS Specialist Nurse – their numbers are rising regularly.

The team approach, although it may have developed differently in different hospitals, is designed to provide a more coordinated approach to the management of MS. Following your initial assessment, team meetings will be held between the professionals, sometimes involving you and/or your family. These meetings lead to the development of a management strategy of MS. The idea is that this should centre on your problems. Sometimes one professional person is appointed to liaise with you, as the first point of contact. Teams may involve the neurologist, a nurse, a physiotherapist, a speech therapist, an occupational therapist, a counsellor, an MS Specialist Nurse and possibly others.

In general, the move to a team approach has been helpful for people with MS, but problems of coordination between the professions still continue to exist, especially in the community. Sometimes you may be somewhat confused by the large number of professional staff you come into contact with. If you can establish one main person for contact – no matter what their professional discipline – it is very helpful. Note that many hospitals are still underfunded, and the team approach in itself will not lead to a change in that aspect, but they might be used more efficiently. In addition, there are often coordination problems between social services departments and other non-health-based support sources.

Visiting your GP/neurologist/MS Specialist Nurse

Getting the most out of your visit

- Ask for an explanation of any words that you don't understand – including illnesses, medicines, symptoms or treatments.
- Ask what results you can expect from any drugs, therapies or medications given to you. Should you expect only a little or a more significant change in your condition? When should these changes occur?
- Ask about any other options that you might have and their advantages or disadvantages.
- Ask about side effects that you might have from any drugs or therapies prescribed for you.

- Ask about any follow-up procedures. When and on what basis will you be seen next time?
- Before a visit to your doctor, write anything down that you need to ask, noting important points that you don't want to forget to discuss.
- Note down important points arising from your discussions with your doctor as soon as possible. Increasingly, some doctors are now happy to allow you to tape record your discussions to jog your memory of what he or she said. Research has shown that having such a recording is a great help to yourself, and your family, in following a doctor's observations or advice.
- Keep a diary of important events or issues between visits to the doctor, so that you can discuss these at your next visit.

Seeing your GP notes

Under recent legislation all patients have the right to see their complete medical notes, and to request corrections to, or deletions of, any inaccurate material – particularly regarding comments on a patient's attitude or state of mind. The doctor is fully entitled to either sit with you whilst you examine the notes or recover reasonable costs of providing copies (including administration costs). However, you can be refused access to notes when there is a reasonable concern that the contents may have an adverse effect on your welfare. Most doctors are very willing to comply graciously with such a request.

Having a check-up

The purpose of the traditional neurological check-up, for which people with MS are asked to return every 6 months or year, is gradually changing. Previously, because there was no real therapy to slow down the course of the disease, the check-up was used to monitor the speed of its progression, and to offer symptomatic and appropriate advice. Many people found this a frustrating system, for often their symptoms were as well controlled as they were likely to be, given the modest resources available, and the consultations following a routine examination frequently appeared cursory, focusing on further decline (or any newly acquired neurological problems) since the last check-up.

However, this approach is changing, as neurologists now turn their attention far more towards assisting people to manage MS medically over the longer term, rather than largely focusing on getting the diagnosis right and seeking confirmation of that through monitoring the disease.

Neurologists now focus far more on what is described as the 'rehabilitative' approach to MS, the battery of newer drugs that might affect the course of MS, and the increasing recognition of the contribution of other professions to your care. All this is changing the 'check-up' process, making it more likely to be of value to you. Often you will be seen by other specialists – perhaps specially trained nurses – as well as the neurologist; thus the increasing use of MS clinics of the drop-in variety is beginning to make the problematic 'check-up' experience of old a matter of the past. However, there are still areas of the country where the old system prevails, and in this case it is very important that you ensure that your questions and concerns are addressed in the consultation with your neurologist – after all it is a two-way discussion.

It is important anyway that some periodic monitoring of your MS is undertaken, to give you further information about likely developments in the disease, and to assess your eligibility for newer drugs, or possibly trials of experimental drugs, that is if you wish to participate. In this case a neurological examination will determine, over the course of time, how many episodes of MS have occurred, how many individual areas of the nervous system have been affected, and the rate at which new areas are being affected. You may also have an MRI scan, which records similar information about changes in plaques, plaque location and severity, but which may, from your point of view, be little related to your symptoms. Your clinical history is also vital when your neurologist is dealing with any new episode of MS that occurs.

Other support

Many people with MS will need professional support services and assistance at some time, to manage the changes in their lifestyles, and to monitor effects of any new drugs. Depending on the precise nature of your MS and its effects, such services may include nursing, physiotherapy, occupational therapy, speech therapy, psychological assessment and support, counselling and advice on housing, employment, financial and other similar issues (see later chapters). Such professional support services for all the many consequences of MS have not previously been adequate, in fact often woefully inadequate and ill coordinated. Despite serious financial constraints, there are now many attempts underway locally to provide better coordinated services and support.

Rehabilitation

'Rehabilitation' is perhaps the new watchword of longer term care in MS. Broadly it means professional care targeted to achieve your maximum potential. Regional Rehabilitation Units have been created in recent years for the support of people with many conditions, but there are also an increasing number of more specialist MS rehabilitation units or programmes. At present there are only a limited number of places available on these rehabilitation programmes, and there is a selection process involved, usually on the basis of who might be expected medically to get the most benefit.

During inpatient rehabilitation you would normally be in a hospital or rehabilitation centre as a patient for some weeks, depending on the programme, your MS and how you progress. In this time you might be offered:

- regular assessment and monitoring of your condition
- carefully targeted drug therapies as appropriate
- intensive physiotherapy and occupational therapy
- nursing care
- possibly speech therapy, and
- psychological and counselling support.

Within a structured programme the aim will be to tailor aspects of this programme to your individual situation and needs. Following the time spent as a patient, you would probably have periodic further assessments to determine how you are progressing. Increasingly MS clinics are being opened in major centres providing support for more people with MS than is available on a lengthy inpatient basis. The aim is to undertake systematic rehabilitation here on an outpatient basis. There is a concern that outpatient care may not be sufficiently intensive to produce major change in functioning.

How useful is rehabilitation?

There is increasing evidence that rehabilitation programmes provide some benefits for people with MS. Studies of rehabilitation programmes are very difficult to undertake in MS for various reasons:

- People have very different types of MS, and it is still unclear as to who would most benefit from the programmes.
- There is no completely standardized programme of rehabilitation.

Studies that have been undertaken so far appear to suggest that a range of benefits arise for many people in the *short to medium term* but, after 1 year or more from the end of an inpatient programme, there is decreasing difference between those who have been through the programme and those who have not. Almost as soon as people with MS are discharged from rehabilitation programmes, they begin gradually to lose the gains that they had from the programme. This is not really surprising because, back home, they do not for the most part have the intensive care available in the programme, and all sorts of other issues intervene to complicate people's lives. This is why there is an increasing emphasis on outpatient care through MS clinics and MS 'drop-in' centres to provide ways of continuing to offer ongoing treatment.

Further studies in this area are being undertaken to see whether there are particular symptoms or abilities that benefit over the longer term more than others from rehabilitation programmes, and which people with MS might benefit most from them.

Going into hospital

Given the range and increasing complexity of tests and treatments, a stay in hospital – even as a day patient –is not uncommon and, if such a stay can be organized over a period of 2 or 3 days, it may be easier for both your neurologist and you to have these undertaken in hospital rather than on an outpatient basis, although outpatient visits will subsequently be necessary. Some treatments are given in hospital. However, neurologists do not agree on how long that hospital stay should be; some feel that the drugs can be administered with very short stays (a matter of hours), while others feel that a day or two to a week, depending on the therapy, may be necessary. Some people with MS may need to go to hospital for investigation of particular symptoms (e.g. urinary problems).

In general, there is very substantial financial pressure, among other issues, to reduce both the number and length of stays in hospital. So, where possible, your hospital stays will be shorter except when you go in for inpatient rehabilitation (see above) and more and more people are given self-injection teaching where necessary.

3

Complementary therapies and MS

When there is no current scientifically accepted cure for a disease, people understandably want to try other means of management. Many people over the last 30 or 40 years have claimed that they have the answer to MS, but the difficult problem for all such potential therapies is to find out whether there really is a connection between the treatment and a remission.

A distinguishing characteristic of complementary therapies is their focus on the 'whole person', using the body's own healing powers. Many of these therapies are only now being scientifically studied. Some complementary therapies fall outside what is considered conventional scientific medicine, but may be used alongside it, such as acupuncture. Other therapies are generally considered much more unorthodox by the medical profession (described as 'alternative'), e.g. naturopathy, herbalism or crystal healing. However, complementary and alternative treatments are often considered as a group under the heading of CAM (complementary and alternative medicines).

Research suggests that up to 60% of people with MS are using some form of CAM – people with MS visit CAM practitioners nearly 50% more often than others without MS. Whilst some people use CAM alone, by far the majority use both CAM and conventional medicine together.

Assessing the value of complementary therapies

There is still a great deal of scepticism amongst many doctors and health professionals about CAM in relation to MS. This is because many CAM therapies have not been fully evaluated using controlled clinical trials – the main way through which conventional medicine is assessed (see Chapter 18). In this situation positive information about CAM is often from CAM practitioners themselves who have a vested interest in their success. Thus people with MS may feel they are caught in the middle, with outright medical scepticism on the one hand, and very partial and enthusiastic support from CAM practitioners on the other hand. Another issue is that many doctors, compared with people with MS, may have very different views and interpretations about the value of CAM therapies in a situation where there is no cure for MS. The way forward, pending more formal assessments of CAM therapies, is to provide as accurate and unbiased information as possible for those who are considering their use.

There are certain key questions that you should ask yourself in relation to any CAM therapy, particularly a new one about which substantial claims are being made:

- What detailed evidence is there that the CAM therapy might help my MS?
- Who has endorsed the therapy? Have leading MS Research Centres or the MS Society supported the use of the therapy?
- What are the possible side effects?
- How expensive is it in relation to the assumed benefits?
- How easy is it to access and undergo?
- Are its practitioners well trained, professionally recognized and insured?
- Would it involve you giving up, or not taking, professional medical advice or treatments?

One of the difficulties for people with MS in relation to many CAM therapies is that, for the most part, they are focused on treating 'the whole person' and on general health, rather than specifically focused on the MS. Thus there is little precise information about any effects on the MS itself. However, as a broad principle, even if the course of your MS is not changed but your general health is improved, this can be helpful in managing your life with MS.

Of course there are many stories about individual cases where a CAM therapy is argued to have dramatically changed the course of MS. Although such stories are very attractive and enticing to people with a condition such as MS, you would be right to be sceptical yourself about whether the CAM therapy itself had caused this change, and even more so about the general effects of such a therapy on all people with MS. You should be very wary about claims of 'miraculous' or 'amazing' results from a CAM therapy. If the claims sound too good to be true, they are just that. Also be concerned about the main evidence for a CAM being given in the form of individual testimonials, rather than through more systematic research. MS is notoriously unpredictable and thus it requires a very careful and controlled study to eliminate any other reasons for a change in the MS.

As a broad guide, the issue for people with MS considering using a CAM therapy is balancing what you consider to be the personal benefits against any side effects and the costs incurred. Realistically it is unlikely that a cure will be found for MS from amongst CAM therapies. However, by feeling better through using them, you may consider that your symptoms have been eased and you feel a lot better about day-to-day living – not least because, unlike many professional staff in the hard-pressed NHS, many complementary therapists have the time to discuss your concerns at length.

A book called *Therapeutic Claims in Multiple Sclerosis* (see Appendix 2) evaluates many therapies proposed for MS. It covers over a hundred different therapies. It has to be said that the evaluation is from a very robust scientific point of view, the evaluations are decisive and usually dismissive on the grounds of lack of scientific evidence for effectiveness. Nevertheless, descriptions of the main aspects of the therapy are helpfully given. A book more sympathetic to the possibilities of CAM therapies in MS, but which is still based on rigorous evaluations, has been written by A. C. Bowling (*Alternative Medicine and Multiple Sclerosis*), and there is an associated website that may be helpful to people with MS (see Appendix 2).

For another sympathetic view of the possible benefits of complementary medicine, you might try the Institute of Complementary Medicine (see Appendix 1), which adopts a very rigorous approach to the evaluation of such therapies, or the individual professional associations of the therapy concerned. This would also enable you to check the qualifications, experience and regulation of their members.

Safety of complementary therapies

Few complementary therapies have been fully scientifically evaluated, especially in relation to MS. Almost any therapy, scientifically evaluated or not, that has the power to produce very good and positive results, has the potential to do harm. Although complementary therapies are considered as 'natural' and, almost by association, to be intrinsically safe, this is not always the case. For example, some herbal medicines have to be very carefully targeted to symptoms and very sensitively administered, otherwise they may be harmful. So it is important both to ask about side effects, i.e. those other than the wanted effects, of complementary therapies, and to be alert in case they occur. Note that practitioners may expect initial 'reactions' or 'aggravations' or symptoms as part of the effective working of the therapy. A competent therapist should both warn you about these and what to do, if and when they occur.

Finding a practitioner

Finding a competent practitioner for a complementary therapy is not always easy. There is little statutory regulation for qualifications or practice for most of the therapies and therapists. However, the best ways of finding a practitioner are through:

- an MS resource or therapy centre, where often other people with MS and staff in the centre will have experience of particular therapists;
- a recommendation or referral from a neurologist, GP or other healthcare professional;
- registers set up by the professional bodies of whichever therapy you are interested in;
- referral for homeopathy to one of the NHS hospitals providing this service;
- contacting the British Complementary Medicine Association, or the Institute of Complementary Medicine (see Appendix 1).

Ask whether practitioners are trained and licensed; whether they are insured for malpractice, negligence or accident; and how complaints are handled. One of the key things is to try and ensure that whichever therapist you go to has a good understanding of MS. Both of you should be able to evaluate its benefits.

Costs involved

Many complementary therapies (acupuncture and osteopathy to name only two) are increasingly recognized as having significant benefits and can, in certain circumstances and limited geographic areas, be made available through the NHS. Many GPs are now more willing to accept and recommend alternatives. However, at present in many cases you will have to pay for your own treatment. The appropriate registration bodies can provide details of registered practitioners in your local area and provide guidance on how much you might expect to pay. You may find the addresses of these registration bodies through the British Complementary Medicine Association or the Institute of Complementary Medicine (see Appendix 1).

Some types of CAM therapy

There are many, many types of CAM therapy that may be used by people with MS, most of which we cannot consider in detail here (see the book by Bowling for more detailed information on individual therapies in Appendix 2). Furthermore the popularity of such therapies in MS can change very rapidly, with new therapies or new variations of previously available therapies regularly appearing, and the use of others decreasing rapidly after only a brief high profile existence. Thus in this section we consider some of the key CAM therapies that appear to have gained longer term use, or appear to be on the verge of doing so.

Cannabis

There has been a great deal of discussion about the use of cannabis recently in relation to the symptoms of MS. Based originally on individual reports by people with MS that at least two of the more problematic symptoms of MS, tremor and spasticity, seemed to respond well to cannabis, there has been an increasing interest in its use by people with MS. However, at present, cannabis is illegal in Britain – some people with MS have already been prosecuted for possessing, growing or supplying it – and it cannot be prescribed for MS.

Nonetheless the pressure from people with MS to research the effects of cannabis more formally has resulted in the setting up of major clinical trials, the most significant of which are funded by the Medical Research Council, although some are being undertaken by pharmaceutical companies. These trials are not using cannabis in its original form, but are using what are called cannabinoids (one or more of the very many active substances in cannabis). Thus if the trials are a success, it will not mean that cannabis itself will be made available to people with MS, but almost certainly will lead to the use of manufactured drugs that have some cannabinoids as constituents. The results of some of the key trials are now beginning to appear indicating that a statistically significant beneficial effect on such MS symptoms as spasticity (and particularly pain associated with such spasticity). In due course one or more products based on such cannabinoids will become available. However, it is important to note that becoming 'available' will almost certainly mean only by prescription from a medical practitioner who is willing to offer such drugs. Furthermore, even then such drugs may not become available through the NHS for some time, and may only be available initially through private payment.

Currently, there is evidence that an increasing number of people with MS are using cannabis on an occasional or sometimes regular basis; it has become a very difficult issue because, although they do feel that they gain from taking it, they are having to balance what they feel is a significant reduction in their symptoms against committing an illegal act. Using the drug in any form is illegal, including 'inactivated' tinctures with limited narcotic effects. Growing, buying, selling and using cannabis carry penalties including heavy fines and jail sentences, even when there may be a medical justification for its use. There is a group campaigning for a change in the law (the Alliance for Cannabis Therapeutics) to allow the use of cannabis for medically designated purposes, and if you feel strongly about the issue you may wish to join this group (see Appendix 1).

Primrose oil

We discuss the role of evening primrose oil in Chapter 10.

Hyperbaric oxygen

Hyperbaric oxygen therapy (HBO) consists of breathing oxygen under high pressure, usually by sitting or lying in a large pressurized chamber, and this proved to be one of the more popular complementary therapies for MS in the 1980s and early 1990s. The former national charity Action for Research in Multiple Sclerosis was instrumental in supporting the installation and running of pressurized chambers in many local therapy centres. A substantial number of these chambers are still in operation in therapy centres now run by Regional Federations of MS Therapy Centres.

The original theory behind the therapy was that MS might be a vascular (blood system-related) condition in which tiny blood vessels in key parts of the nervous system become blocked by fatty globules circulating in the blood, thus leading to nervous system damage. It was thought that hyperbaric chambers (used to assist the management of nitrogen 'bubbles' in the blood of divers suffering from the 'bends'), might be a way of eliminating these circulating fatty globules, and perhaps – through the use of additional oxygen under pressure – might even repair existing damage. Many people claimed success in managing symptoms, and even slowing down or stopping the course of their MS. However, clinical trials of HBO produced a much less promising outcome. HBO did seem to have an effect for some people in lessening urinary symptoms (such as incontinence) and in reducing fatigue, but had no significant effect on any other symptoms, or on the course of the disease. Many people who say that they feel better as a result of HBO still use the therapy, although most doctors are very sceptical that it has any real effect on MS.

Whether you choose to have HBO is, of course, up to you. The main issue from a personal point of view is setting the benefits that you feel you may be obtaining against the practical issues of attending a centre on a regular, often initially daily, basis, and being in a chamber for an hour or more while it is pressurized, reaches its appropriate 'diving depth' and then depressurized. Costs for HBO in the therapy centres are often subsidised, but can still be relatively expensive over the initial phase of the therapy.

Herbal products

Although we often think of herbal medicines as being 'alternative', in fact a high proportion of both over-the-counter and prescribed drugs have a plant origin. However, in recent years, herbal medicine, often considered as a natural non-manufactured therapy, has become very popular. Practitioners operate under a range of different approaches. Although herbal remedies sound very benign and safe, they can be very powerful and can have side effects. Make sure that any practitioner is very well trained in the properties, toxic as well as beneficial, of the herbs that are used, and also has a good knowledge of MS. Herbal medicine and its practitioners are amongst the newest professionalized groups engaging in complementary medicine, even though herbalism has a very ancient history. Many herbal products available in chemists and health food shops, are capitalizing on the popularity of herbal approaches to health.

A detailed overview of the possible effects of the many hundreds of individual herbal products on MS is beyond the scope of this book, and indeed good herbal practitioners would argue that a careful process of individual diagnosis and therapeutic recommendation is needed for someone with MS. However, there are some general guidelines that it is helpful to bear in mind:

- It is wise to think of herbs in the same way that you think of drugs (indeed many herbs are drugs).

- Many herbs contain compounds that have not yet been fully identified, and some of these may be toxic.
- Good preparation of herbal medicines is critical to ensure both their safety and their efficacy.
- Be very careful when using herbal medicines if you have several medical problems, or are pregnant or breastfeeding.

Some herbal medicines interact with proprietary drugs often used to treat MS or its symptoms, so it is particularly important that you talk to your doctor first if you are taking such drugs.

As with other complementary therapies, certain herbal remedies may be of value in relation to general health, and certain symptoms of MS might indeed be helped, but there is no evidence that herbal medicine can alter the course of MS. As a final warning, it is worth noting that some Chinese herbal remedies may contain animal products, of which some may be from banned sources, or not included on the label. For a more detailed review of particular herbal products in relation to MS, see the relevant section in the book by Bowling (see Appendix 2).

Homeopathy

Homeopathy is a system of therapy in which minute doses of a substance are taken on the basis that these will cure or control symptoms that would be produced by the very same substance in much larger doses. This is often described as an approach where 'like cures like', which some people argue is similar to that of vaccination, where a very, very small dose of a disease may protect against subsequent infection – although in the case of homeopathy, the small dose is to remedy what is seen as a current 'disease'. It is argued that, paradoxically in relation to conventional science, the smaller the dose the more powerful the effect. Many scientists argue that the doses are so small that they cannot be detected using laboratory instruments and are thus sceptical about the efficacy of homeopathy, but homeopaths believe that their system of therapy is both effective and safe.

Homeopaths normally focus on the person as much as the disease, and thus any specific symptoms of MS are only one aspect of the person's life and experiences, used to determine a relevant therapy. As the homeopathy is undertaken on such a person-centred basis, it has proved difficult to undertake clinical trials to prove to the scientific community that it is an effective help for people with MS. Increasingly more sophisticated trials are being developed, and some have shown that homeopathic preparations do have a statistically significant effect on certain symptoms, although not yet in relation to MS. Nevertheless, there are people who claim that homeopathic treatment has substantially helped their symptoms. As might be anticipated from homeopathic theories, if a remedy is given that appears to be relevant to the symptom, an initial 'aggravation' of the symptom may occur – in short it can get worse – before any improvement is noticed.

Acupuncture/acupressure

Some people with MS have reported some benefits from either acupuncture or acupressure. Acupuncture, in its traditional form, is based on the idea that energy (*chi* or *qi*) flows round the body through channels (called 'meridians'), which become blocked at times of illness and stress. Acupuncturists use the insertion of very fine needles at key points on these meridians unblocking energy flows to help restore health. Acupressure (often known as *shiatzu*) works on a similar principle, but uses pressure from fingers or thumbs at these energy points.

As with some of the other complementary therapies, it is difficult to undertake a scientific trial of the value of acupuncture or acupressure, although some very specific testing has been undertaken on pain and nausea relief using particular acupuncture points. The results suggest that, in certain circumstances, acupuncture does appear to relieve pain and nausea; however, it would be wise to seek a diagnosis of why you have pain or nausea from your GP or neurologist, before undertaking such a treatment for pain, in case there are other causes that need to be treated, or indeed other ways of relieving the pain that may be more effective.

There have been some, albeit small, and uncontrolled studies of acupuncture on people with MS. Reports from these studies indicated a range of mild benefits in relation to several symptoms, which suggests that larger and better conducted studies should be undertaken. Acupuncture may have some effects on the immune system, although this has not yet been fully explored. However, it should be noted that, although acupuncture is generally extremely well tolerated, there are occasional reports of pain and soreness at the needle site, as well as stiffness and muscle spasms. This may be due both to skin sensitivity, and a tendency to muscle spasms in MS.

Yoga

Yoga is widely used by many people with MS, and there are now both specialist centres and teachers for them. From a practical point of view, in many respects yoga can be seen as providing a form of exercise known to be helpful in keeping your muscles working, as well as providing a form of calming of the mind, helpful in countering depression, stress and fatigue. Yoga is also a form of meditation that requires dedication and time. For those people who can commit to it, it may help not only with individual problems (such as work-related stress), but also everyday living. For some people it can lead to a more rewarding lifestyle. In some circumstances yoga may prove an effective technique for the management of individual symptoms (such as stress or pain), but you will benefit largely from your own efforts.

One advantage of yoga for people with MS is that, in addition to its emphasis on slow movement, and peace and calm, once you have received some training, you can undertake the exercises at home, without any additional equipment or expense. Its emphasis on deep and controlled breathing can also be helpful, particularly if your posture is not what it should be, or if you are sitting for long periods. The main concern with yoga and MS is that you should work well within your limitations in a relaxed way, and be careful not to push yourself too far, or raise your body temperature, as this may increase fatigue. If you are undergoing, or have been undergoing physiotherapy, it may be an idea to consult your physiotherapist before starting yoga.

You can obtain more information about yoga from the Yoga for Health Foundation, which runs special classes for people with MS and other conditions, or from the Yoga Therapy Centre at the Royal London Homeopathic Trust (see Appendix 1).

Massage

There are many forms of massage. Some of them are very vigorous and seek to realign any muscles of the body that the therapists believe are out of line. Such forms of massage should be avoided by people with MS, for many of the problems faced by people with the disease, such as spasticity, are a result of neurological damage, and cannot just be 'reworked' by a very vigorous massage. The more relaxing and gentle forms of massage, on the other hand, are potentially of considerable value, not only in relaxing muscles and reducing spasticity, but also in promoting a general sense of wellbeing. It is very important that you check what form of massage the therapist is offering, and ensure that the therapist has been well trained and, above all, knows about MS.

Aromatherapy

Aromatherapy is usually a massage with essential oils; sometimes oils are heated and released into the atmosphere around you. Although, in other forms of massage, an oil is often used as a lubricant during the massage, in aromatherapy specific oils are used for massage or heating and release, following an aromatherapy diagnosis of your state of mind and body. The oils are very concentrated, and should always be used in a carrier oil (such as sweet almond oil) during massage. They must not be taken by mouth. Some of the oils should not be used if you are pregnant, or have certain other conditions, such as epilepsy, and it is crucial that you let your aromatherapist know about these. Although some of the more exotic and far-reaching claims for aromatherapy have never been tested, some people with MS have found it very relaxing and stress-reducing.

Reflexology

Reflexology is a therapy based on the idea that energy and other flows in the body are linked to, indeed terminate, at key points in the feet, providing a 'map' of key organs and systems in the body. It is believed that problems in all areas of the body can thus be identified and indeed treated through manipulation of the feet.

Some people with MS have indicated that they have found this therapy helpful and relaxing, although there is no formal evidence that it affects the course of MS, or even major symptoms of the disease. However, as a relaxing therapy, it may benefit some people with the condition.

Chiropractic

Chiropractic is a long-standing approach to health based on a particular view of the ways in which the human body works and may be managed. Practitioners manipulate the bones, muscles and tissues, especially around the spine, to enhance health. In chiropractic, the focus is mainly the nervous system, and enhancing the blood supply around key tissues. Practitioners can use a variety of techniques, which vary in strength.

Chiropractic is founded on the belief that a wide range of bodily pain and disease processes originate in abnormal nerve function. A course of treatment is usually composed of short sessions spaced out over several months. Treatment consists of manipulation of the spinal column and individual vertebrae. Chiropractic recommends itself particularly for back pain and persistent headaches. In very rare instances, manipulation of the spinal column can cause lasting damage, so always ensure that you consult a qualified chiropractor and that you discuss your MS fully before any treatment begins. It is increasingly likely that your own doctor will know more about chiropractic and can discuss any possible benefits or disadvantages with you.

Osteopathy

Osteopathy is a relatively well-regulated and trained profession compared to other complementary therapies, and a practitioner must be registered with the General Council and Register of Osteopaths (see Appendix 1). Osteopathy, like chiropractic, is a long-standing approach to health in which practitioners manipulate the bones, joints, muscles and tissues, especially around the spine, to enhance health. In fact osteopathy regards the entire musculoskeletal system as the critical basis of good, and ill, health. Treatment may involve established medical diagnostic procedures (including X-rays and standard biochemical tests) in addition to manipulation of joints, rhythmic exercise and stretching. Osteopathy can improve mobility in some affected joints. Cranial osteopathy involves gentle manipulation of the bones of the head and spine.

The main concern, as with the other complementary therapies, is the extent to which the use of osteopathy could significantly affect the course of symptoms of MS. Whilst a sense of wellbeing may well result from its use, there is no evidence that it has any effect on the course of MS itself.

As a concluding point, it is important that you take note of what your physiotherapist says about osteopathic or chiropractic treatment, particularly if he or she has wide experience of people with MS, has been treating you for some time, and knows your own situation well. In addition, if you feel that your physiotherapy is helping you manage your MS, then there is every reason to stick with it – particularly as you will almost certainly have to pay additional money for osteopathic or chiropractic diagnosis and treatment. However, some people with MS have found such massage to be of value, but it is not possible to know whether you will be one of these people.

Meditation and relaxation techniques

'Mind and body' alternative therapies have become increasingly popular in relation to MS in recent years. The rationale of such therapies is that, if a state of mental relaxation can be achieved, anxiety is decreased, and beneficial physical effects will occur – such as muscle relaxation and reduced blood pressure. There are many different techniques for achieving such mental relaxation. Indeed there are many different meditation techniques some of which are relatively simple to undertake; others require much more training and support.

As far as MS is concerned, particularly in improving muscle relaxation, meditation and relaxation techniques may help reduce the incidence of muscle spasms and spasticity. At a more general level there is an increasing but under-researched possibility that relaxation techniques may improve the operation of the immune system. In general the possible benefits can be set positively against what, is for the most part, a very low-cost alternative therapy.

4

Problems with urination and bowels

Urinary and bowel function problems probably cause the most inconvenience to a person with MS. They can be embarrassing to cope with and may be the ones most difficult to discuss with your doctor. As such symptoms in MS are likely to result from damage to the spinal cord, they may also be associated with sexual dysfunction as well as other symptoms such as weakness and spasticity.

Bladder control

This is one of the most difficult issues to deal with in MS, despite being a very common symptom. Research has suggested that between 80–90% of people with MS have urinary problems of some kind, although they vary widely in type and seriousness. More expertise and resources are now being devoted to dealing with it.

If particular nerves in the spinal cord are damaged by MS, then urinary control will be affected. There are several kinds of urinary control in people with MS that might then be affected:

- They may urinate involuntarily – either just dribbling a little, or sometimes even more (a problem of 'incontinence').
- They may wish to urinate immediately (a problem of 'urgency').
- People may wish to urinate more often than before (a problem of frequency). When people have frequency at night, i.e. needing to urinate several times during the night, it is called 'nocturia'.
- They may fail to empty their bladder (a problem of 'voiding').
- They may find it difficult to begin to, or to continue to urinate (a problem of 'hesitancy').

The major bladder problems in MS can be summarized as either:

- a failure to store
- a failure to empty, or
- a combination of both.

In general the more serious the MS, the more serious your urinary symptoms are likely to be. About 65% of people with urinary problems have difficulties with urgency, or frequency and incontinence resulting from urgency. About 25% have difficulties in relation to urine retention and bladder emptying, and the remaining 10% may have both sets of problems.

Whilst many of the common urinary problems above that people with MS experience are indeed a result of damage to the nervous system caused by the disease, others may be caused by 'urinary tract infections'. Urinary tract infections are not caused directly by the MS itself, but are more likely in people with MS because of some of its functional effects – for example through infections from a failure to empty the bladder. Thus it is very important that you are regularly tested for urinary infections. This is particularly important if the bladder problems you have are significant.

Diagnosing a bladder problem in MS

The most helpful information for a doctor or other health professional to assist in diagnosing your problems is a brief history of any bladder symptoms you may have, for example:

- What is your major concern about your bladder/urination?
- How often do you urinate during the day/night?
- Do you leak when you laugh, or cough, or do you have an accident? How often? In what circumstances?
- Do you find it hard to begin urinating? Do you feel that you empty your bladder?
- Do you wear pads or protection? If so how often?
- When and how often have you had kidney infections?
- Do you have pain on urinating or blood in your urine?
- Have you had any formal investigations before, or are you taking any medications?

If responses to these questions suggest the existence of bladder problems, then it is likely that you will asked to take some tests.

Tests

Increasingly there are different tests being used to determine more accurately what the exact problem is. Your GP will probably only undertake tests for urinary tract infections, and it will be your neurologist who may refer you to specialists, e.g. a urologist, for other tests, if necessary. The two most significant tests assess:

- urinary tract infection, and
- control of urinary flow.

Tests for urinary tract infection. Doctors are recognizing that urinary tract infections are an increasing problem for people with MS and often associated with retention of urine in the bladder. However, it is important that you ask your doctor to undertake such tests regularly. If your doctor suspects that an infection is present, a 'mid-flow' sample of your urine is normally requested and, after the specimen has been 'cultured' to identify the particular bacteria present, you will be prescribed the most appropriate antibiotic.

Tests for urinary flow. More and more sophisticated tests, known as 'urodynamic' tests, are being developed to measure 'urinary flow'. A more recent test investigates this flow and the amount of urine remaining in the bladder after urination by taking a non-invasive ultrasound picture of your bladder. Of particular importance is the measurement of the amount of urine remaining in the bladder after you have urinated – it is this residue that can give rise to infection. This overall test, called an 'ultrasound cystodynogram' (USCD), is gradually replacing one that measures the rate of flow or urine by the introduction of a 'catheter' (a thin tube) through your urethra (the opening in your body from where urination occurs) to your bladder. The remaining urine then flows out and can be measured. To obtain additional information, further ultrasound pictures might be taken of your kidneys. Very occasionally, a far more intrusive investigation – 'cystometry' – is performed, usually only in very rare cases indeed, to allow the examination of the inside of your bladder (almost as a final resort after all other methods have been tried with no success), and when surgery is being considered. Surgery is rarely, however, considered for urinary problems in MS, for it is often associated with a range of side effects and difficulties.

Managing urinary symptoms

The management of urinary symptoms can take various forms, depending on the diagnosis of the problem. In most cases initially this can result in a combination of strategies including:

- lifestyle changes (changing your everyday routines)
- specific exercises and bladder training

- using a continence product (e.g. absorbent pads) occasionally or regularly
- taking appropriate prescribed drugs.

In relation to more serious urinary symptoms, additional measures may be necessary including:

- catheterization – either intermittent self-catheterization, or on occasions a more permanent indwelling catheter
- surgical intervention.

Problems of frequency and urgency

These are two of the most troubling symptoms for people with MS. The issue of urinary urgency, often combined with wanting to urinate more frequently is one of the most difficult problems for people with MS earlier in the disease. It is usually caused by the bladder not storing the urine properly, or a lack of coordination between the storage and emptying process. It is wise to plan ahead whenever you leave home, and ensure that there are always toilet facilities within easy reach, but there are other aids.

As a self-management technique, pelvic floor exercises help to tone the muscles in and around your urinary system. This is sometimes called 'bladder squeezing' and helps to decrease frequency and urgency problems in some people. As a general rule, exercising your pelvic floor muscles is a very good idea, although other help may well be required. If the frequency and urgency continues to be a problem, which they may well do so, you may have to turn to drugs.

In effect many of the drugs which are used 'slow' the bladder by decreasing the transmissions to the nerves causing the bladder to empty. Oxybutin chloride (Ditropan) is an 'anticholinergic' drug that, in effect, blocks the nerve signals that trigger the muscles to release urine. This can be very effective, but is also associated with side effects, such as a dry mouth, because the drug blocks the nerve signals to the salivary glands as well. Indeed, without a dry mouth, it may be that the dose is too low. Unfortunately, you may become constipated, and at very high doses there may be problems with your sight. Often you have to experiment under the guidance of your doctor to find the most appropriate dose level controlling frequency and urgency with minimal other side effects. Another anticholinergic drug, propantheline, can be used, although trials have shown it to be slightly less effective than oxybutin. An antidepressant such as imipramine (Tofranil) may also be prescribed – not for depression, but because it has been found to have an effect in controlling urgency.

More recently, a drug called capsaicin – derived from red chilli peppers – has been found effective in people with MS with relatively serious incontinence, who might find the side effects of the anticholinergic drugs unacceptable. Although this drug is still under evaluation for long-term safety and effectiveness, it appears to provide good control for quite long periods of time, i.e. 3 or 4 months from one administration usually in a hospital. It is not yet widely available, and it appears initially to make symptoms worse rather than better, before it takes full effect. So some people have to be 'catheterized' (see below) for the first few days after the administration. So far, people who have used it have found it sufficiently beneficial to come back for further administrations of the drug. Other natural products like ginger have also been tried. There is a vast amount of information on the internet that can be perused, but many of the studies have not been proven scientifically.

You may not need to take one of these drugs continuously, but you could use it for a particularly important event or journey when you need to avoid urinating for some time. For peace of mind on particular occasions, you could use a protective pad to absorb urine, in case you have 'an accident'. As a final point, people who have urinary problems often also have mobility problems – the nerves controlling both legs and the urinary system are situated close together – so the difficulties experienced through frequency and urgency are often compounded.

Nocturia

Another problematic symptom for many people with MS is that they may have to get up to urinate several times in the night. Nocturia, as this problem is known, is quite common. The usual medication for nocturia is desmopressin (DDAVP Nasal Spray) which reduces urine formation. There are some circumstances where the drug should be used only very cautiously, or not at all – for example, in people with kidney or heart disease, or in older people. The antidepressant, imipramine (Tofranil), mentioned above in relation to treating urgency and frequency, taken just before going to bed, has also been found to be effective in many cases.

Incontinence

Incontinence, what appears to be the involuntary release of urine, may be a slight and an occasional problem in MS, or it may prove to be a continuous problem. However, in each case it provokes anxiety and concern, for socially as much as physically it can be a difficult and embarrassing symptom to have occur unexpectedly. This can be caused by a number of separate problems. Bladder spasms may be causing this difficulty – technically called 'incontinence' – or your bladder muscle may be so weak that you have released urine before realizing it. In addition, sometimes you might not at first realize that you are wet because of reduced sensations in your pubic area.

The first step where minor and occasional incontinence is concerned is, as a means of 'insurance', to use a protective pad. Sanitary protection (absorbent pads) can be used, even if only for maintaining confidence when you are not near a convenient toilet. Pads and liners are available in a wide variety of shapes and styles to suit different people and different clothing styles, but there is much less choice when they are supplied on prescription. Waterproof undersheets and absorbent bed sheets can also be very convenient, to minimize the effect of occasional accidents.

If these procedures and/or the drugs mentioned above in relation to urgency and frequency do not work, other professional investigations may well be needed to determine the cause of the problems, and how best they might be managed.

Catheterization

Although your major concern may be incontinence, there may also a problem with urine retention in the bladder as well – for the bladder may not completely empty, which can lead to serious infection. Thus as an extra precaution, if one of the causes of the incontinence is retention of urine in your bladder, the use of 'intermittent self-catheterization' (ISC)

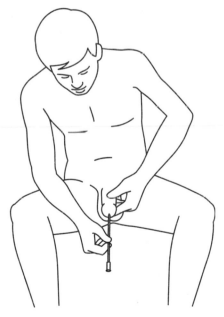

Figure 4.1 Self-catheterization.

might help (Figure 4.1). ISC is used to ensure that the retained urine is regularly voided. Although you can do it yourself, a carer can also help you. A catheter (a thin plastic tube) is threaded through your urethra – the opening at tip of the penis, or just above the vagina – into your bladder, and this drains any remaining urine. You will need to wash yourself thoroughly before using this technique, and you may need to use a lubricant (something like K-Y Jelly) to assist the access of the tube, but modern catheters are low friction types and need no lubricant (such as 'Lofric' and 'Speedicath' types). You withdraw the catheter as the urine begins to stop. You should not use a catheter (tube) which appears to be worn, stiff or damaged in any way. You can do it while sitting on the toilet, or lying down. Undertaken regularly, several times a day, this method usually helps substantially. A nurse or doctor will explain how to undertake this procedure, and how to clean the catheter thoroughly. For the most part, although the procedure may seem very difficult, many people adapt well to it, as long as it is seen as a routine process. If you are able to write and to feed yourself, even if you have some eyesight problems, ISC should be possible. There is another reason why ISC can be of value, in that regularly undertaken, it is a means of 'training' the bladder to fill and empty as the urine is released: the bladder muscle contracts, expanding again as urine fills the bladder.

Urine retention and voiding problems

As we have noted above, many people with MS have problems not only with urgency or frequency, but also with some urine retention in the bladder. If this is the case, do not reduce your fluid intake substantially, because this will increase the risk of urinary infection (urine as a waste product is not being diluted). A useful rule of thumb is the colour of your urine: if it is dark yellow to brown in colour, then almost certainly you are not taking in enough fluid.

There are some useful guidelines which should help you:

- Drink at least 2 litres (or just over 3 pints) of liquid a day.
- In general, an acid urine helps keep infections at bay.
- Decrease your intake of citrus fruits/juices.
- Foods and substances that neutralize acidity, including antacid preparations, such as sodium bicarbonate, should be eaten less often, as should dried vegetables.
- Increase your intake of proteins.
- Drink cranberry juice, and eat plums and prunes regularly. Cranberry juice will also help to provide the vitamin C lost through reducing the intake of citrus fruits/juices.

Hesitancy and 'full bladder' feeling

Although this is a frustrating problem, often urination will start after a couple of minutes, so be patient! Sometimes tapping very lightly on your lower abdomen – but not too hard – will help; this often produces a reflex reaction of urination.

There have recently been trials of a hand-held vibrating device which, when held against your lower abdomen if you are still sensitive in this area, seems to work quite well by increasing urinary flow and leaving less urine in your bladder. It is probably most useful for people with relatively mild MS.

Of course, other time-honoured techniques may work, including turning a tap on and hearing the sound of running water! A more direct method is to stimulate the urethra gently, at the tip of the penis or just above the vagina, with a clean finger or damp tissue.

If you have the feeling that your bladder is still full, this may need further investigation. It is important that your bladder is as empty as possible after you have urinated, not least to try and avoid an infection. Intermittent self-catheterization (ISC) may help, as may anticholinergic drugs. If you need further advice, make an appointment to see your doctor or, if possible, your neurologist or continence nurse/advisor.

Urinary tract infection

If urination is painful or associated with a burning sensation, and even more so if it smells unpleasant and is cloudy, the chances are that you have a urinary infection. In this case seek medical advice as soon as possible. In the meantime you should try and increase your fluid intake.

Kidney infections are particularly worrying in MS: they may be associated with both abdominal pain and a high fever, and require a tougher drug approach, perhaps with intravenous antibiotics. The problem is that, once infections get a hold in the kidneys, there is a substantial risk that they pass unchecked into the bloodstream, and cause major, even on occasions life-threatening, difficulties. You may also experience increased frequency and urgency with an infection. On the other hand some urinary infections in MS can be almost symptomless, and thus periodically – and especially if you feel that you suffer from some problems of urine retention – ask your doctor if you could have a urine test for infections just to make sure.

For people who seem particularly liable to urinary tract infections, a long-term low-dose antibiotic might be given occasionally to eliminate or suppress bacteria.

General precautionary steps to prevent bladder infection could include:

- Attempting to empty to bladder as often as possible – holding urine in the bladder for long periods should be avoided.
- Women should be careful to wipe from front to back and to avoid underclothes made of synthetic materials, which can trap infection. It is also a wise precaution to empty your bladder both before and after sexual intercourse.
- You need to ensure that you take adequate amounts of fluid (see above).
- You might also consider taking substantial does of vitamin C because this will make your urine more acid and less liable to bacterial growth.

Indwelling catheterization

When urinary difficulties become a real problem, a permanent catheter can be fitted. Although some may think this is more convenient, it is not an easy step to take for many others; some actually think of it as the hidden equivalent of being in a wheelchair. Furthermore, medically, it is best if some other way can be found to manage urinary problems. An indwelling catheter opens up the inside of the body to the continual possibility of infections from which it is normally protected, even during ISC, and it can be particularly dangerous if you have a weakened immune system. Therefore, in principle, the less time that people with MS use an indwelling catheter, the better. If the MS becomes more severe, there may be no option, particularly when you cannot undertake ISC, or when drugs or other strategies do not appear to deal with the problem.

How it works. An indwelling catheter can be inserted through the urethra (like ISC), or through a specially constructed surgical opening in the lower abdomen, above the pubic bones ('suprapubic catheterization'). Whichever route is chosen, the catheter is inserted into the bladder, and then a small attached balloon is inflated (which you won't feel) and filled with sterile water in the bladder itself. Through the other end, on the outside of the body, urine is continuously drained into a collection bag.

Increasingly, the medical preference is to insert the catheter through the special opening in the lower abdomen. This is because a permanent catheter through the urethra may enlarge, change or disrupt the urethral opening, and make it difficult to maintain control of the urine. An indwelling catheter like this can cause problems with sexual activity and we deal with this elsewhere in Chapter 5. Even if a catheter is inserted through the lower abdomen, there are still likely to be some problems:

- Infection can occur around the site of the insertion.
- The catheter can periodically become blocked.
- The catheter needs to be changed every few weeks, and sometimes more frequently.
- Kidney stones can form.
- Catheters can sometimes become detached or loosened and thus require monitoring; this has to be done by someone else if your MS is severe.

It is important to increase fluid intake if you have an indwelling catheter to help prevent infections – these occur more frequently if you don't drink enough.

An indwelling catheter can be used on a temporary basis, or for particular occasions when other means of urinary control are difficult, but you need to discuss all this with your doctor or continence nurse. Each insertion runs a risk of introducing infection and it has to be undertaken as meticulously as possible.

Surgery and urinary problems in MS

Surgery is very rarely performed to ensure urinary control in MS – indeed it seems to offer no major improvement in such control. Several procedures are possible, but are only undertaken on rare occasions when almost all else has failed, and a more or less intractable problem remains. There is another factor here: MS, over time, is a progressive disease, and it is possible that once you have undergone some surgery, other surgical procedures may then be needed later, to manage further problems that might arise.

Other management techniques

In addition to trials of further drugs that may be of value to people with MS, some other procedures or techniques may help. Research has suggested that **bladder training** – involving working out a schedule of regular urination on the basis of ultrasound assessments – together with ISC, may be helpful. Because of the association between CNS control of leg function and urinary function, an appropriate **exercise regime** may help the urinary function indirectly.

Bladder training generally involves a series of educational and training exercises. It is important to note that some substances such as caffeine and alcohol can cause additional urgency with frequency, as can one of the common artificial sweeteners – Nutrasweet. Eliminating these products may help substantially. Training may involve you resisting or trying to slow down the urge to urinate so that urination can be undertaken more on a kind of timetable, perhaps every 1–2 hours. Urination can also be partly controlled by how and when drinks are taken.

Electrical stimulation of various kinds comes into vogue from time to time to help with urinary control. A few of these techniques, some of which use small portable instruments, may prove to be of some value:

- TENS (transcutaneous electrical nerve stimulation)
- DSCS (dorsal spinal cord stimulation)
- ESES (epidural spinal electrostimulation), and
- SES (spinal electrostimulation).

There is considerable energy being devoted to developing and testing some of these procedures. All these can be discussed with your continence nurse.

Related problems

For most younger people (those in their 50s and below), the urinary symptoms caused by MS will probably be far more significant than those arising from other causes, and thus the focus should mainly be on these. However, there are some circumstances that may be associated with an increased likelihood of urinary problems.

Men and prostate problems

As men get older, some have problems from prostate gland enlargement. This gland surrounds the neck of the bladder and the beginning of the urethra. By the age of 60, it is enlarged in some 60% of men, and the proportion increases even more with age. Very often, the symptoms of an enlarged prostate develop slowly, but as they can echo some urinary symptoms caused by MS – particularly increased urinary frequency, urgency and nocturia – it may be difficult to separate the causes without investigation. As with other symptoms, it is important that specific causes are found, if possible, so that they can be appropriately managed. As the life expectancy of people with MS increases, more men may find that an enlarged prostate gland makes some of their urinary symptoms worse.

Childbirth

Recent research has also shown that urinary problems may occur earlier in life for some women following a difficult or problematic childbirth. The control of urination is a frequent minor problem following childbirth. It is not clear how such problems interact with those of MS. However, many techniques of management indicated in this section can be used, although it would be wise for women who feel their pregnancy and childbirth has affected their bladder control to seek professional help and advice.

Bowel function

Even for people without MS, constipation is a very common problem, as evidenced by the number of remedies available in chemist shops, but there are some special issues that may make constipation worse, more frequent, more continuous or, indeed, more problematic for people with MS.

Until a few years ago problems with bowel function were thought to be relatively minor; however, recent research studies, as well as the views of people with MS, have clearly indicated that these can be a real problem. The most common issue is constipation – that is infrequent, incomplete or difficult bowel movements. There may also difficulties with bowel urgency, where there is a need to pass a stool immediately or urgently, or with bowel incontinence, where control of defaecation is effectively reduced or lost.

Constipation

Constipation is problematic in MS because it can make other symptoms, such as spasticity and urinary difficulties, worse as well as producing pain or discomfort. Constipation may result from several causes in MS:

- Demyelination may reduce the speed with which the movement passes through the bowel; as moisture is drawn from the stool continuously, the lower the speed, the more the movement becomes dry and hard and difficult to pass.
- You may have decreased sensation in your bowel or rectal area thus not realizing that a bowel movement is needed, and therefore the stool is left in your bowel for a very long time.
- You may have too low a fluid intake thus making the stool dry and hard.
- You may have weakened those muscles that push the stool out and thus have difficulty in this respect.
- In some cases drugs for other symptoms or for the MS itself may affect either the dryness of the stool, or the capacity to push it out.

When MS becomes more severe, it is much more likely that people with the disease will have difficulty evacuating their bowels, as various body systems linked to this process become less efficient. You may need to undergo detailed medical investigation and get help for this problem.

For most people with MS who have constipation, especially in the earlier stages of the disease, the advice is very similar to that for other people with the same problem. In particular:

- Your diet should be high in fibre (e.g. bran, cereals, fruit and vegetables), which allows stools to pass more easily through the intestinal tract.
- Fluid intake should also be increased for the same reason.
- Getting as much exercise as possible can help, although clearly this particular advice will be less easy to follow by those who are bed-bound or using wheelchairs. In this latter case seek advice from your physiotherapist.
- Proprietary bulking agents (such as Fibogel, Metamucil, Mucasil), and stool softeners, can help produce regular motions.
- You could use laxatives, suppositories or enemas occasionally if all else fails, but be careful about using any of these too regularly, because they can actually increase constipation if overused, by slowing down natural bowel function still further.
- Finally, make time for regular daily bowel habits (see below).

As medical and related products are often readily available and may be recommended by some to deal with various problems associated with constipation, it is important to describe briefly some of these products.

- **Bulk formers.** These are useful when there is inadequate bulk in the motion. They add moisture and content to the stool. The bulk formers should be taken with a couple of glasses of water. They distend the gastrointestinal tract making the passage of stools easier. Motions should pass through in a day or so after their use. Bulk formers are not habit forming and can be used regularly.
- **Stool softeners.** If the cause of the constipation is a hard stool, which is difficult to pass, then a stool softener can draw increasing moisture into the stool from body tissues therefore softening it and helping elimination. Again these are not habit forming and can be used regularly
- **Laxatives.** These should be used only occasionally; they are not only very habit forming, but also lead to a weakening of the remaining muscular control of the bowel. Harsh laxatives in particular should be avoided, because basically they are chemical irritants of the bowel tract. Softer laxatives, which should only be taken occasionally, can lead to passing motions in 10–12 hours.

- **Suppositories.** These, placed in the rectum, both provide chemical stimulation and lubrication. They may be used occasionally to stimulate a bowel movement.
- **Enemas.** These should be used only very occasionally because the bowel may become dependent on them if they are used frequently.

You may have to be patient to try and find the right combination of strategies that works for you. It is likely that a successful overall strategy will consist of a good fluid intake, a diet with high fibre, as much exercise as possible, and a regular time for a bowel movement – 30 minutes after a meal is usually the most opportune time.

Faecal incontinence

This has been a neglected area in MS. Recent research has revealed that something like two-thirds of people with MS have some bowel problems and, over several months, nearly half, in one study, had some degree of what is described as 'faecal' or 'bowel incontinence'. Of course, what appears to be an involuntary release of faeces produces a very unpleasant situation. There may be a link between urinary and bowel incontinence (from weakened muscles, from spasms in the intestinal area induced by MS, or from a full bowel pressing on the bladder), but the link is not always clear.

The exact causes of bowel incontinence are not always easy to find, even in the few centres with special facilities for investigating these issues, but there are several pointers to what may be happening in many cases. Involuntary spasms in the muscles affecting the bowel area are probably the most common causes of such incontinence. Sensation may be reduced in the bowel area and you may not be aware that there has been a build-up of faecal material, until an involuntary movement of the anal sphincter occurs. Prior constipation might lead to this build-up and release of faecal material, as well as a lack of coordination in the muscles controlling bowel movements.

There are a number of ways in which the problems of faecal incontinence may be helped. It is important to ensure that you have bowel movements (and thus bowel evacuation) on a regular basis. You should avoid substances that irritate the bowels such as alcohol, caffeine, spicy foods, and any other triggers to involuntary bowel action that you can identify. For such a symptom, antibiotics may be a trigger, thus you need to avoid their unnecessary use. It is also important to eliminate the possibility that the faecal incontinence is caused by a bowel infection – to test for this possibility you will need to consult your doctor.

Spasms

Stabbing pains in your midriff may be caused by 'bowel' or 'colon spasms'. These are due to either MS directly or changes in bowel function and regularity. Changes in diet and supplementary bulking agents may be all that is required to deal with this problem. If it persists, then antispasmodic drugs may calm your bowel or colon. (See also the section on *Pain* in Chapter 6, and *Diet and nutrition* in Chapter 10.)

Management techniques

Although constipation and bowel incontinence may look like two separate problems, often they may be linked, so initially it is a good idea to try similar management. This involves establishing what is often known technically as a 'bowel regimen'. In addition to checking your diet, making a regular time of day in which you try and have a bowel movement can be very helpful. Once this regular time is established, it is important that you stick to it – even though you may not feel the urge to go. You may find that drinking some warm liquid, such as tea, coffee or water, will help. This 'retraining' is not an easy task and may take some weeks or even months to achieve, but there is some evidence that it can reduce both constipation and bowel incontinence.

You can undergo some complex tests for difficult problems with bowel incontinence, but there are still relatively few specialist centres to assess and help manage these problems. Thus for most people with MS, a tried and tested combination of everyday techniques will probably be a good first step.

5
Sexual relationships

Many people are diagnosed with MS at a time when they are, or may be about to become, sexually active in their relationships. The issues associated with how best to manage sexual activity and MS have in the past often proved difficult to discuss with others. However, increasingly, both doctors and other health professionals concerned with MS are aware of the importance of such issues and are able to offer helpful support and advice. In this chapter, we address some of the common worries that men and women with MS, and their partners, may have. *Multiple sclerosis – the 'at your fingertips' guide* contains more information on this subject. We start with a discussion about problems with erections, common issues affecting men with MS, and their sexual relationships.

Problems for women

In general women's sexual problems are centred on a lack of desire, arousal and orgasm. Lack of desire is the chief complaint among women. A woman's lack of sexual interest is often tied to her relationship with her partner. It can also be triggered by family concerns, illness or death, financial or job worries, childcare responsibilities, managing a career and children, previous or current physical and emotional abuse, fatigue and depression – as well as by the MS itself. Thus the issue is often trying to deal with a range of factors in managing sexual problems. Nonetheless there is a particular set of problems that may occur as a result of the MS, particularly centred on arousal, and subsequent problems of lubrication.

The process of sexual arousal is similar in women to that in men: in women the engorgement of the sexual organs (the clitoris and the inner and outer labia round the vagina), and lubrication by internal secretions, occur. For many women such a process is not just an aid to sexual intercourse, but also a considerable aid to sexual pleasure. In MS

nervous system control of the process of engorgement is likely to fail –
parallel to the process of erection in men. Furthermore, sensations in the
breast and genital area may be also affected.

The usual – and it must be said – still relatively common view in such
circumstances is that artificial lubrication, through the use of a
lubricant such as K-Y Jelly, is sufficient to deal with problems such as
vaginal dryness but, whilst such lubrication can help sexual intercourse,
it may well not deal with the complex range of other issues that
surround sexual arousal and fulfilment in women.

Exercises for women

Although there are several possible causes of your loss of sexual drive,
and thus several possible approaches to managing the difficulty, as far
as some of the physical components are concerned, the female orgasm
involves – amongst other things – the contraction of several sets of
muscles around the vagina. There is increasing evidence that exercising
these muscles can assist in providing the conditions for better sexual
responsiveness. Relevant exercises involve periodically squeezing and
then releasing the pubococcygeus muscle – the one that starts and
stops urination in mid flow – several times a day if possible. This can
help tone the muscles, and possibly enhance vaginal sensations, which
may help responsiveness.

If you have no partner, or indeed wish to attempt to do something
yourself to enhance your sexual life, then there are a range of things you
might try, including the use of fantasy, or sexually explicit books or
magazines, and physical exploration of yourself. Some women use
vibrators to provide additional physical stimulation. Although it is
difficult to create sexual sensations to order, using one or other of these
might help you to regain some of your libido – even if this requires more
imagination than usual! Remember that some women without MS do
not have perfect and completely satisfying sexual lives!

Viagra, Cialis and Levitra for women

In principle, these drugs could help to enhance sexual pleasure by
promoting the engorgement of the clitoris and the inner and outer labia.
Until relatively recently, although there are reports of individual women
who have found Viagra helpful, there have been few systematic studies of
women's sexual response using the drug, and none in relation to women
with MS. Women may feel that this again shows very particular gender
priorities in the testing of such drugs.

However, although a number of studies show that women tend to report more sexual problems then men, there is less evidence that a drug such as Viagra will assist with many of their problems. By and large, the major problems for many women are concerned with desire and arousal, rather than with the engorgement of their sexual organs alone. In particular, as it has been graphically put, often 'the most important sex organ for women is between the ears, not in the genitals'. Thus it is not at all clear that many women as might be expected will be helped by the physical effects of such drugs alone, although it is important to note, for some women with MS in particular, the local genital effects of such a drug might be beneficial when there are difficulties, for example, with lubrication. Nonetheless many drug companies over the last two years or so have begun the development and testing of drugs, which potentially may have a range of effects on women's sexual desire, in addition to similar effects to those of Viagra.

Difficulties with erections

First, it may be helpful just to explain a little of the 'mechanics' of an erection. The penis is made up of the 'urethra', which runs through it and carries both urine from the bladder and semen from the testes, and which is surrounded by the 'prostate gland'. On the underside of the penis, and running along its length, is a mass of spongy tissue called the corpus spongiosum. Alongside this spongy tissue are two 'chambers' called the 'corpora cavernosa' in which millions of tiny pockets fill up with blood during an erection. Special cells in the penis limit the flow of blood into these pockets most of the time, for otherwise there would be a perpetual erection! When these special cells 'relax', they allow the pockets to fill with blood, and thus the penis becomes erect, and when they 'contract' the blood is expelled and the erection subsides. A range of enzymes and other chemical substances work together to facilitate blood flow into and out of the penis.

Erections may not occur, either because of vascular problems, i.e. problems in the blood supply to penis, or, and much more likely in MS, problems in the control of erections through the nervous system, which controls the process of erection and ejaculation.

Managing erectile problems in principle involves attempting to deal with the problems in the nervous system; dealing with problems in the vascular system, and in addition dealing with psychological and related issues. For many men with MS with erectile problems, drugs like Viagra have appeared to provide an immediate and helpful way forward.

Viagra and other help for erections

The introduction of Viagra was a breakthrough in the management of erection problems. Two more drugs, Cialis and Levitra, have now been added to the options available. It is important to explain how this type of drug works. They do not repair any of the nervous system damage caused by MS. Essentially they act on the vascular problems in MS, by assisting the penis to fill with blood. They do this by breaking down an enzyme (a chemical messenger in the blood) that is preventing or seriously slowing down the process of engorgement of the penis. By magnifying the effectiveness of the erectile process, even where this was previously weak or virtually non-existent, erections can be maintained as long as the drug effect lasts. These drugs may be able to help such problems in many men with MS; indeed, there is very strong evidence that men with erection difficulties caused by MS are likely to benefit from them.

At present they are taken orally (by mouth) and, because of the relatively slow digestive process, it may be an hour or two before the drugs produce their effects – certainly an issue in planning sexual activity. Viagra, Cialis and Levitra affect not just the penile area, but have potential effects all over the body, so there may be some side effects elsewhere. Your cardiovascular health will be carefully assessed before they are prescribed. Not everyone will benefit, although firmer, more frequent and longer lasting erections have been found in two-thirds to four-fifths of men who used Viagra.

Because the drugs are costly, and the demand is assumed to be large, the Department of Health has been extremely circumspect about those who can be prescribed them. However, MS is now one of the designated medical conditions by the Department of Health for which these drugs can be prescribed, and so there should be fewer difficulties in obtaining them on these grounds, although there may still be local variations in supply plus, of course, any clinical reasons for their non-prescription.

Currently there are a number of other drugs under development, which promise similar overall effectiveness to that of Viagra, but with a greater immediacy and convenience of use. In particular the aim has been to ensure as far as possible that spontaneity can be preserved in relation to sexual activities. The forms in which Viagra can be used are also being developed and before long there will be several different ways in which it can be administered.

Side effects

With the publicity for these drugs have come reports of some potentially dangerous and unpredictable effects. We need to clarify the position.

We have already noted that they work on the vascular system. Most reports have centred on vascular incidents, such as deaths from heart attacks. There are several points that need to be made here. In the population at large, impotence and erection problems increase with age, and so statistically much of the demand has come from older men. However, cardiovascular problems – heart disease and high blood pressure – also increase with age. Although these drugs have been found to enhance erectile function in those with such problems, men who are taking medications such as organic nitrates, which reduce blood pressure, e.g. nitroglycerin (trade names Nitro-bid, Nitrostat), isosorbide dinitrate (trade names Isordil, Sorbitrate), pentaerythritol tetranitrate (trade names Penitrol, Peritrate), and erythrityl tetranitrate (trade name Cardilate), may well suffer a dangerous further drop in blood pressure by taking such drugs. Such medications are also likely to be prescribed more to older men. In addition, and a rather obvious point, sexual activity, and particularly sexual intercourse, involves vigorous exercise, and men who have undertaken almost no exercise for several years, perhaps with an underlying undiagnosed cardiac problem, may find themselves in difficulty – as in undertaking any vigorous activity without prior preparation. The doctor prescribing these drugs will understand these problems. However, because many men with MS are in younger age groups than those in which major problems have occurred, it is likely that the difficulties will be found to be fewer amongst most men with MS.

Other help available

Even if the nerve pathways from the brain to the penis are damaged in the middle or upper parts of the spinal cord, the pathways in the lower part of the spinal cord may still be intact. If this is the case, stimulating your penis directly, most helpfully with a vibrator, could result in an erection. You could also induce an erection by placing the (non-erect) penis in your partner's well-lubricated vagina – with your partner sitting astride you. However, it is important that this is undertaken carefully, for if sensation levels are low, your penis might be damaged by being folded over, without this problem or any subsequent injury, being realized at the time.

There are a range of devices used in treating men's erectile problems, although many of them are now being replaced with Viagra or other related drugs, because they are less intrusive and more effective.

Vacuum pumps

The least intrusive of these options is the vacuum pump, which should be available to you on prescription. A tube is placed over the flaccid penis, sealed at the bottom round the base of the penis, and air is pumped out either manually or by a battery-operated pump. This causes blood to enter the penis and for it to become erect. A band is then slipped from the bottom of the pump around the bottom of the penis, the pump removed and the penis then stays erect with the blood trapped inside. It is important not to keep the band round the base of the penis for longer than 30 minutes, and the placing of the band round the bottom of the penis may require some dexterity.

Injections, prostheses and aids

Other more intrusive forms of erectile assistance include penile injections that relax the smooth muscle normally inhibiting blood flow into the penis, thus allowing an erection; or penile prostheses that can be inserted surgically that allow an erection to take place with various forms of mechanical assistance.

There are a wide range of issues and concerns relating to the use of penile injections and prostheses, and both require an exceedingly well-organized and planned approach to sexual activity, and intercourse in particular, which some have found difficult to reconcile with anticipated emotions and feelings. If Viagra, Cialis or Levitra are not available, then you should seek a referral from your GP or neurologist to a physician specializing in these other techniques.

There are also a number of artificial aids that do not require medical consultation or prescription, and these may include latex or similar penises, some of which are hollow and can incorporate a flaccid penis. Vibrators and other aids in the form of a penis are also available in sex shops or by mail order.

Psychological problems and 'libido'

Depression or fatigue, which are indirect (or secondary) symptoms of MS, may play as large a part in the way that you feel sexually as does primary neurological damage. If such symptoms are treated successfully, then your sexual drive (often called your libido) may increase.

If the primary cause of your decreasing sexual drive lies in primary neurological damage, then this is harder to deal with directly. You and your partner could consider first sensual activity experiences, without you feeling the immediate pressure for sexual intercourse. Some parts of your body will probably be more sensitive than others. Ensure that you make time to enjoy the experiences with each other without feeling hurried or under pressure. As in other relationships where circumstances change, new, and possibly exciting and stimulating, patterns of mutual exploration may need to be learnt or re-learnt.

Problems during intercourse

Incontinence

If you haven't had one already, visit your doctor for an assessment of the problems you have with incontinence. Try and ensure that you have no urinary infections, which can make your bladder problems worse if left untreated.

The following advice can help reduce the risk of 'accidents' during intercourse:

- Reduce your intake of fluids for an hour or two beforehand.
- If you are self-catheterizing, do so shortly before you begin.
- If you are taking drugs to reduce urgency because of a bladder storage problem, take these about 30 minutes beforehand to ensure as far as possible that no spontaneous bladder contractions occur.
- You may need to ensure more vaginal lubrication, with something such as K-Y Jelly.
- Check out gently and sensitively positions in which you both feel comfortable, and in which you feel you are less likely to have problems with leakage.
- If the woman has an indwelling catheter, then several positions may be better than others (remember also to empty the collecting bag, and tape the catheter to prevent it moving): a rear entry position may be easiest to manage, lying on your sides with the man behind; or, while the man kneels, the woman could lie on her back with her legs over his shoulders.
- Alternatively if the man kneels and, as it were, sits on his knees with the woman in front of him with her legs over his shoulders, then gentle movements in this position should be more comfortable. If the woman has problems with spasticity in her legs, then such a position is likely to reduce the possibility of annoying cramps and rigidity.
- The male partner could use a condom, which might be useful for other reasons as well.

Pain

Low levels of sexual arousal can reduce lubrication in the woman, but it can also be due to damage to nerve pathways in the mid- and upper spinal cord area, which leads to inadequate stimulation of the lower nerve pathways to the genital area; certain drugs taken for other purposes – such as urinary problems – also dry up vaginal secretions. Sometimes lubrication can be helped by direct stimulation of the genital area; or try to set up an environment which is relaxing and conducive to sexual thoughts and experiences. As far as additional lubrication is concerned, K-Y Jelly or a similar water-soluble substance can be very helpful. Substances like Vaseline are not recommended because they do not dissolve in water, and they are likely to leave residues which could give rise to infections. They can also create holes and tears in condoms.

Spasticity

Check with your doctor that the general control of your spasticity is as good as it can be. Try and keep your muscles as well toned as possible through regular exercises (see Chapter 8), and use appropriate drugs such as baclofen as necessary to give additional control.

There are also certain positions for sexual activity that appear to make the muscular spasms less likely, although it is important that you explore other possibilities than those mentioned below, for you may find another position that suits you both very well. For a man who may have difficulty with spasms or rigidity in his legs, then sitting in an appropriate chair (without arms) would allow his partner to sit on his penis either facing him or with her back to him. For a woman, lying on her side may help, perhaps with a towel or other material between your legs for more comfort. Your partner can then approach you from behind. Another possibility is to lie on your back towards the edge of your bed with the lower part of your legs hanging loosely off the bed.

Fatigue

As with other symptoms associated with MS, it is important to discuss this with your doctor who will assess the best means of managing it. Although there are one or two drugs which may help (for example amantadine or pemoline) and which – if prescribed for you – might be taken a few minutes before sexual activity, currently the best help is through various appropriate lifestyle changes. The use of various techniques to assist with fatigue is discussed in more detail in Chapter 7.

Consider when you feel least fatigued. Although this may not necessarily be the time when you feel that you should be having sex – such as in the morning, or during the day, rather than at a more conventional time – you may be less tired and enjoy it more. Rather than thinking of sexual intercourse as the major element, you could agree with your partner to engage in some other less energetic sexual activities – such as gentle stroking or foreplay – that you could participate in more frequently. As with so many other aspects of living with MS, it is a question of finding ways to adapt to the situation through experimentation.

6
Sensations and pain

Of course, not every twinge, or pain, results from the MS. When you visit your doctor, particularly your GP, you may find that he or she puts virtually all your symptoms down to MS itself. Whilst statistically it is probably correct that most of your symptoms **will** be related to the MS, many **will not**. It is easy for both of you to say 'Oh, that's another symptom of MS' and not realize that, like other people, you can have other everyday problems. It is important that both are recognized in relation to pain as well as other symptoms.

If GPs do confuse MS and non-MS symptoms, this is not through incompetence – even specialists sometimes have similar problems. Most GPs have so few people with MS on their patient lists – often only one or two – that, because of all the other pressing demands on their time, they have not been able to study, and experience, all the many twists and turns of the disease. Try a little persistence if you feel that your symptoms are not being treated as carefully as you wish; you can always ask for a second opinion if necessary.

Sensations

Initially strange and sometimes uncomfortable sensations of many kinds are typical effects of MS. A person can feel these symptoms but the doctor may to be able to find clear physical evidence of why particular symptoms are caused. They are related to damage to the nervous system. They may take various forms, and are frequently intermittent. Doctors often regard these symptoms as *relatively* benign because, although they may be irritating, they do not, on the whole, tend to result in major problems in daily functioning. Many people with MS get to know the situations in which these sensations occur and adjust their everyday lives as much as possible to avoid those situations. Some may be uncomfortable but can be tolerated. Others may be helped by remedies that you can use yourself. Yet others may require medical advice, support and treatment.

It is often felt by doctors that, although it is now recognized that pain is more frequent and often more severe than previously thought, it does not generally lead to decreased mobility, and is not associated with a poor prognosis. This may offer some comfort to those who have pain from their MS.

'Burning'

A burning pain can occur in your arms, legs and in other parts of your body. Medically, this is often called 'dysaesthesia' and results from abnormalities in the sensory pathways in the nervous system. After exercise, or at night, this burning pain may get worse. Unfortunately, ordinary pain medications do not usually have much effect on this kind of sensation. Antidepressant medications such as amitriptyline may be used for relief if it becomes too problematic, or other remedies, such as antiepileptic drugs (gabapentin and carbamazepine), may be used to try and alter conduction along the nerve fibres, which has produced the sensation.

'Pins and needles'

MS affects many nerve pathways in the CNS, and those related to sensations in the body are particularly prone to damage. Depending on where the damage occurs, you may feel all sorts of unusual sensations in those areas. The sensation of pins and needles commonly occurs with the interruption and resumption of nerve signals to particular areas of the body. Closely related sensations, such as **tingling**, may also appear occasionally, as signals to and from the affected area vary. Some clinicians treat this symptom as relatively unimportant, albeit a disconcerting, symptom of MS, for it has generally a less direct effect on everyday activities than 'motor (movement) symptoms', and is associated with a slower course of MS. As with the burning sensation, there is no specific drug therapy for such symptoms although, if the symptoms are associated with pain, a tricyclic antidepressant or sometimes medications such as carbamazepine and valproic acid (usually given for antiepileptic purposes) can help.

Trembling

Most people have some kind of 'tremor' (or trembling), albeit slight, as there are several different types. Your limbs will normally be the parts affected, as the course of the disease progresses. The most common is what is known as **action tremor**, although it can be described as **intention tremor, goal-directed tremor**, or **hyperkinetic tremor**. This is caused by damage to the nerve pathways to the balance centre of the brain. The nearer your hand approaches an object when reaching for it, the more your hand trembles, so it then becomes difficult either to pick up or control something like a cup. Other kinds of tremor are much rarer.

As there are no specific drugs for the treatment of action tremor, doctors tend to try a range of different ones in the hope that one or other may prove of benefit, but it is difficult to avoid unwanted effects. Drugs known as beta-blockers, such as propranolol, might help. People often tend to develop ways of helping themselves. These include such things as:

- bracing an arm against a piece of furniture;
- making the arm immobile for a specific task;
- working out movements with a physiotherapist that are as smooth as possible;
- adding weights to an arm, using weighted utensils such as forks and spoons.

A far more drastic approach to reduce action tremor is through surgery, but currently this operation carries considerable risks of exacerbating other problems, and could make life worse, not better, for you. Various newer surgical procedures to control tremor are under development, including the implantation of electrodes, but many of these are still only experimental and, in any case, may only be useful for a small group of people with MS.

Numbness

Numbness is quite a common and upsetting symptom in MS, although it can be only temporary if you have a relapse. There may be other strange and sometimes unpleasant skin-based sensations. Usually the worst of these will 'wear off' relatively quickly, although they may stay for days and sometimes longer. Because sensory nerves, in various parts of the CNS, link to all parts of your body, inflammation or damage to them can produce numbness almost anywhere, but particularly in your feet, hands, limbs or face. You may think the nerve damage has occurred where the numbness is; in fact the damage will be in the CNS, often well away from where the symptom appears. Numbness in the hands can cause difficulties for holding or picking things up, particularly those that are hot or sharp. Check carefully where and how you are walking, if the numbness affects your legs.

Even though depression may not be present, again tricyclic anti-depressants can help to reduce the feeling of persistent numbness, and intravenous steroids can be used when the numbness is, or appears to be, associated with a relapse.

Sensations and heat

The extent to which the symptoms of MS appear to change with temperature differences has been known for a long time. In fact, with what seems now to be extraordinary insensitivity, people with suspected MS used to undergo the 'hot bath' test, in which they were given a hot bath. If their symptoms became worse, this was thought to indicate that MS was indeed a possible diagnosis.

Heat, particularly enhanced body heat, changes the process of nerve conduction, and may result in the sensation of weak muscles and limbs. Heat can also exacerbate other symptoms, such as pain associated with inefficient nerve transmission. Conversely, when the core body temperature is cooler, nerve conduction and muscle function appear to be better, particularly in MS. In general, therefore, people with MS are right to try and avoid situations where their core body temperature is raised.

Tests have been made on body cooling systems, which could be used to maintain a lower body temperature in hot conditions, or more generally to improve the performance of a person with MS in many different temperature ranges. Other approaches to the problem have been more limited and functional: the use of cold or frozen gel packs held in special vests, so that working or undertaking other activities in hot conditions does not raise your body temperature to any great degree.

Balance

Socially and physically loss of balance is a difficult issue to manage. Unfortunately, there is no easy solution, as the loss of balance is basically a problem caused by damage to part of the brain – the 'cerebellum' (or its pathways in the brain stem). Other factors can compound the problem, such as spasticity or weakness in the legs. After a while you will probably adjust to some of your problems and, although you may wish to keep going for as long as possible, the most obvious way of helping yourself is by using walking aids (perhaps a stick or crutches); at least these will help you avoid some painful falls and also signal to others that you are not drunk, but that you have some physical problems with movement.

Dizziness

Dizziness (if due to true 'vertigo') is when you feel that things around you are moving, or feel that you are moving, sometimes quite rapidly, when in reality neither is happening. This can sometimes be alarming, especially if you feel that you are falling. Sometimes other sensations, like feeling sick ('nausea'), are associated with vertigo. Dizziness from loss of balance is also related to damage to the cerebellum (or brain stem), the nerve connections to it from the middle ear, or within what is called the 'vestibular system of the inner ear'. In almost all cases in MS, the dizziness goes away of its own accord after a few hours or days.

Dizziness can be helped by some drugs:

- Steroids (particularly intravenous methylprednisolone) can help when the dizziness is both acute and persistent.
- Diazepam (Valium) is given to dampen down the reflexes of the vestibular system.
- Antihistamines can provide some help if the symptoms of vertigo or dizziness are mild.
- Stemetil (prochlorperazine) may be prescribed.

There is one other apparently strange method that people use: when the vertigo feels worse on moving, exaggerating those movements can sometimes help. Deliberately falling on to a bed (or other very soft surface) on your left and right side, and backwards, three times each way, may 'rebalance' the vestibular system, at least temporarily. You may also find that there is a particular position that lessens the vertigo, such as lying on one side rather than another. There is also some evidence that tolerance can develop (e.g. dizziness can be lessened) if you can, with professional help, maintain the position of your head, when the dizziness is at its worst, for as long as possible. Of course, this approach can be rather uncomfortable until tolerance increases.

Pain

For many years MS was considered, medically, to be a painless disease, probably because the process of demyelination was thought in itself not to be painful. However, people with MS themselves have known for many years that specific symptoms could cause considerable pain, and this is now being recognized.

Chronic pain is experienced by about 50% of people with MS. Although pain is more common amongst people with severe MS, and amongst older people with the disease, almost everyone will experience some kind of pain at some point.

Trigeminal neuralgia

Trigeminal neuralgia is a very acute knife-like pain, usually in one cheek, and sometimes over one eye, but it rarely affects both sides of the face. It is caused by the lesions of MS damaging trigeminal nerve pathways. Drug treatment usually includes carbamazepine (Tegretol), although this drug does produce side effects, which may be a problem. The primary side effect is sleepiness, so the drug may be started in low doses and then given in higher doses until the pain is controlled. It is also possible that phenytoin, which has a milder action than that of carbamazepine, may be used, or less commonly, baclofen, which is usually given for spasticity. Another approach is to try and block the inflammation; if this is associated with a relapse, steroid therapy is given. If there is a continual problem of trigeminal neuralgia linked to several relapses, then a prostaglandin analogue called misoprostal (Cytotec) can bring relief. In some cases, various surgical operations, including the 'gamma knife', can destroy the relevant nerve pathways. Even if the trigeminal neuralgia reappears, as it can do, then the treatment can be started again, and it will almost certainly reduce the pain.

Jaw pain

There are other types of pain that may affect the facial area, which may not be linked to particular forms of myelin damage: temporomandibular joint (TMJ) pain affects the jaw area, or you may get more general migraine or tension headaches. Drug therapy can help counteract this pain, but in each case will be dependent on a careful investigation of the cause of the pain, and particularly the extent to which it appears to be linked to the MS, or to something else.

Pain from unusual posture and walking patterns

Pain from poor posture when sitting or lying, and from unusual walking patterns, is quite common. In most cases the pain does not result from the neurological damage of MS, but from its effects on movement.

In fact one of the most common kinds of pain treated by neurologists in relation to MS is low back pain, often arising from an abnormal sitting posture or from a way of walking that has developed as a result of damage to the control of leg muscles. This may result in a pinched nerve from 'slipped discs', or other back problems, which can also be caused by unusual turning or bending motions. Painful muscle spasms may also result.

So it is important to pay careful attention to how you sit and how you move in order to lessen such difficulties. You may need to seek advice from a physiotherapist in relation to both posture and movement. Comfort may be obtained by:

- massage of the back, if carefully undertaken
- ultrasound
- TENS
- specific exercises, to relieve muscle spasms
- drugs designed to reduce spasms, and finally
- surgery, if there are disc problems.

Other painful conditions, particularly painful swelling of the knee(s) or ankle(s), can result through problematic patterns of walking. You must seek careful advice in relation to these conditions. It is possible that orthopaedic doctors, recommending conventional orthopaedic exercises for such conditions, may not fully realize that having MS could mean that such exercises fail to work. It is likely that the swelling/pain of one joint may be easier to remedy through what is called an 'assistive device' (e.g. a crutch) to take the weight off a weaker leg, or a knee brace.

Spasticity and pain

Muscular cramps and spasms are known as 'spasticity'. Several muscles contract simultaneously, both those assisting movement and those normally countering it. These muscles will feel very tense and inflexible – this is because what is medically called their 'tone' increases, and movement becomes more difficult, less smooth and possibly rather 'jerky'.

Spasticity is quite a common symptom in MS and is often very painful: it can occur in the calf, thigh or buttock area, as well as the arms and, occasionally, the lower back. Spasticity can lead to 'contractures', where the muscle shortens, making disability worse.

There are a number of ways of managing spasticity in MS:

- Use your muscles as much as possible in everyday activities, and undertake regular stretching exercises to help reduce muscle shortening.
- Specific exercise recommended by a physiotherapist, such as swimming, or undertaking stretching exercises in a pool-based

environment, should be done on a **regular** basis – an important point, as spasticity is likely to be a continuing issue.

Devices to assist in the management of spasticity

There are specific devices that may be useful for people with MS when spasticity occurs regularly in key muscle groups, and exercises alone do not appear to deal with the problem. There are devices to spread the fingers or toes. What are called 'orthoses' – in effect braces – keep the hand, wrist or foot in an appropriate position or prevent ranges of movement that may result from, or cause, spasticity. A particularly useful brace may be one that places the ankle in a good position in relation to the foot (called an ankle–foot orthosis – see also Chapter 8) and thus lessens the possibility of local muscle contractures, as well as lessening the stress on the knee. It is important that all orthoses are specifically suitable for the individual concerned, as of course body shapes and sizes vary considerably.

Drugs

There are several drugs available to help muscles relax, and ensure that as few of your activities as possible are affected. It is difficult to target spasticity specifically, so some people may need medication occasionally, in the day or at night, and others may require more continuous medication. It is difficult to get the balance and the dose right, and this often has to be done on a trial and error basis.

One of the most common and effective drugs for spasticity is baclofen (Lioresal), but it can have side effects; some people find it hard to tolerate high doses. Effective doses may vary widely for different individuals. Normally this drug is taken by mouth, but other ways of administration are being developed to help people with more severe symptoms.

Other muscle relaxants, such as the widely used diazepam (Valium) can also be used, but they may have general sedative effects, causing drowsiness; this is why diazepam might be particularly helpful at night. People are also worried about whether they might become dependent on these drugs in the longer term.

There are some newer drugs in the process of being introduced, which on their own, or in combination with the more established drugs, may target the spasticity more specifically:

- Dantrolene (Dantrium) tends to reveal and possibly exacerbate any muscle weakness that may be present, and its effects should be carefully monitored.

- Tizanidine (Zanaflex) is a relatively new drug, and may work in some cases when baclofen and other drugs do not; it can also be used in conjunction with baclofen. It produces more sedation than baclofen but less weakness.

Some other drugs work best for specific muscle groups in the body – such as cyclobenzaprine HCl, which is useful for the back muscles, although it may work for other muscle groups as well. It can also be used in relation to another drug for spasticity.

In relation to chronic spasms, which may result in a complete arm or leg being extended or stiff, carbamazepine may be used, although baclofen can be very helpful. Cortisone can sometimes be used to assist short-term control of such spasms – although it is not for long-term use because it has a range of side effects.

It is possible that any or all of the drugs above may become less effective over time and thus one of the possibilities is to stop taking the drug concerned for a period of time before starting it again.

There are other drugs undergoing trials at present in relation to the control of spasticity. One of the most promising is cannabis (or, in practice, combinations of cannabinoids – the chemical constituents of cannabis). We discuss the present position in relation to cannabis in Chapter 3.

There may be occasions, especially later in the course of MS, when treatment needs to be more robust to reduce very severe spasticity. This might take the form of injections, directly into the nerve or muscle concerned, with phenol or alcohol or, more recently, botulinum toxin, which damages the nerve and produces what some call a 'nerve block' preventing the spasticity from occurring.

Spasticity and surgery

Surgical intervention may be tried in relation to spasticity if other means of control fail. This can take several forms. Nerves controlling the specific muscles of the leg may be deactivated using what is called a 'phenol motor point block'. This may make the legs more comfortable but clearly does not assist mobility. Other techniques may help spasms in the face – indeed botulinum toxin (Botox), which is increasingly being used for cosmetic purposes, may help small but very irritating facial spasms. Sometimes nerves or tendons controlling specific muscles that are producing major problems might be cut if there are no other easy means of control.

A relatively recent development is the use of baclofen pumps to deliver the drug directly into the spinal canal to control spasticity. This process is still expensive and is what doctors would call an 'aggressive' treatment for spasticity, although it does allow a much finer and more detailed management of the flow of the drug.

Pain from other MS symptoms

Apart from the types of pain that we have already discussed, there are other sorts that can be associated with MS symptoms, such as that from:

- urinary retention or infection;
- pressure sores (later on in the disease), if not treated as early as they should be;
- eye conditions, especially 'optic neuritis' (see Chapter 11), when the optic nerve swells.

In general, if the source of the problem is treated, the pain will disappear, although the management of the neurological causes of pain is more difficult than management of pain from other sources.

7
Fatigue, cognitive problems and depression

Until a few years ago, the symptoms associated with MS that we discuss in this chapter were often ignored or underplayed by doctors and neurologists. This was, in part, because MS was considered then to produce mainly – often only – physical symptoms directly (and obviously) related to the damage occurring in the nervous system. Other symptoms seemed – at the time – to be very difficult to relate to nervous system damage in this way, so fatigue, cognitive problems and, to a substantial degree, depression, were often seen as not related to the disease process itself. There has been a very substantial change over the last decade and now much greater professional attention is being paid to people who have these symptoms.

Fatigue

Fatigue or tiredness is one of the most debilitating symptoms of MS and one that worries many people. Up to 90% of people with MS experience overwhelming tiredness at least some of the time. Fatigue in MS is often associated with:

- heat (or being hot) (see Chapter 6);
- activity – using motor skills, or being mobile;
- sleep disturbances;
- particular mood states (such as depression – see later section);
- some cognitive problems that may occur in MS (see later section).

At present there is no one known cause of fatigue in MS. Some argue that the best way to manage fatigue is to consider it as a symptom arising from several different sources and thus requiring different techniques to manage it. In fact it might rather better to talk of 'MS fatigues' in the plural. We could distinguish what we might call:

- **normal fatigue** resulting from everyday exertion etc., which is managed by rest;
- **'MS fatigue'**, which seems to result from the MS itself and for which it is difficult to find any other immediate cause, and which may well require drugs to control it;
- **muscle fatigue**, which may appear in an arm or leg, for example after or during a walk; rest may be needed and cooling may be helpful here;
- **fatigue from depression**, often managed through the treatment of the depression itself;
- **fatigue from drugs themselves**, occurring as a side effect – being aware of this possibility should prompt you to consult your doctor if fatigue seems to be related to a drug you have taken;
- **fatigue from the underuse of muscles** – just as fatigue can result from overuse, it can also result from underuse, it is important to keep your muscles in the best condition you can.
- **fatigue from managing MS** – living with MS is fatiguing for most people, so pacing your activities as well as taking advantage of as many helpful pieces of equipment as possible will be important;
- **fatigue from loss of sleep** – this is of course a problem not just for people with MS and will compound other kinds of fatigue, so the reasons you are losing sleep need to be addressed.

Management of fatigue

Although it is important that your symptom is recognized as genuine by medical and other healthcare staff (which has been a problem in the past), you will probably have to manage many of the day-to-day aspects of fatigue yourself, for drug therapies (see below) are often only partially successful.

Self-help

- Identify activities that appear to precede the fatigue and avoid them whenever possible.
- Develop 'pacing' strategies, trying to work intermittently with rest periods, or use some other ways of relaxing during the day.
- When the fatigue seems to be related to particular times of the day, focus your activities at other times.
- Try longer term 'pacing' too, trying to balance activities over periods of days or weeks.

People with MS may do something that they enjoy or indeed have to do, knowing that they will have a couple of 'bad fatigue days' following this activity. However, 'fatigue management strategy' tends to be a complicated business, taking a lot of energy in itself to think through all the possibilities that might occur.

Professional support

Specific and carefully planned exercise programmes have been found to reduce feelings of fatigue, but only temporarily. Behavioural therapy can help to alleviate other psychological symptoms that might exacerbate the fatigue, but these non-drug professional approaches have not been successful so far for most people with MS over the medium and longer term.

Drugs

Some drugs have helped, the two most well known being magnesium pemoline (Cylert), which stimulates the CNS, and amantadine hydrochloride (amantadine; Symmetrel), an antiviral agent. It has also been suggested that fluoxetine (Prozac) may help in managing MS fatigue.

Some antidepressants, particularly those that have a low sedative effect, may help the tiredness even if you are not clinically depressed. Beta-interferon drugs may have some effect on fatigue if, indeed, they help the immune system.

Fatigue may be one thing that affects cognition, although it is still not yet clear exactly how this happens. Some people with MS feel fatigued almost simultaneously as they notice problems with their memory or concentration (see below). Self-rated fatigue is linked with certain forms of memory problems, as well as reading comprehension. However, if fatigue is treated with a prescribed drug, it does not appear to influence cognition. In order to try and understand this process, fatigue in people with MS has been compared to that in people with chronic fatigue syndrome (CFS), but it is not clear whether the two are the same; indeed, when fatigue severity is the same between the two groups, people with MS showed more widespread cognitive problems.

Cognitive problems

Research has identified two broad areas where MS seems to be involved or has effects that are not so much to do with the mind in general, but with what are more neatly and technically considered as cognitive issues on the one hand, and attitudinal and emotional issues on the other.

Cognitive issues are those that concern our thinking, memory and other skills, which we use to form and understand language; how we learn and remember things; how we process information; how we plan and carry out tasks; how we recognize objects, and how we calculate. It was thought until recently that memory loss and some other cognitive problems were a rare occurrence. However, more recent research has suggested that a range of cognitive problems varying widely in type and severity may be present in many people with MS.

Of course people with MS, just like anyone else of a similar age and sex, can suffer mental illness or dementia but, clinically, people with MS do appear to have more depression (see next section) compared to other people, and perhaps have what might be called mood swings rather more often. More recently, studies have shown that many people with MS have some problems with memory and with what are called their cognitive abilities, and these seem to be associated with the effects of the disease. It is thought that MS could lead to a subcortical dementia but this is not inevitable. We discuss depression and mood swings later in this chapter.

How to recognize the problem

We can all change without necessarily realizing the nature or extent of that change – until someone tells us. Sometimes people with MS may be so depressed or anxious that they think their cognitive problems are worse than in fact they are; on the other hand, they may not want to acknowledge them at all, for they do not want to think that MS may affect their cognitive as well as their physical functions. In addition to the general variability of symptoms, an issue that we have indicated is characteristic of MS, we have also noted that previously it has been very difficult to link cognitive performance to any other aspect of MS. However, more recently, studies using MRI (magnetic resonance imaging) have shown that the more general the demyelination the more likely it is that significant cognitive problems will also exist. Moreover, MS lesions in certain areas of the brain seem to be associated with cognitive difficulties. Further work will, it is hoped, be able to identify more precisely the relationship between certain kinds of cognitive problems and areas of the brain affected by MS.

In addition, during acute attacks of MS, it has been observed that cognitive performance – memory and concentration, for example – may get significantly worse and then improve again; on the other hand, if the cognitive problems have arisen gradually and have been present for some time, then it is unlikely that they will improve substantially.

Family perceptions may be more accurate on occasions but, although we all suffer from memory lapses from time to time, it may be tempting for you or some family members to put down every piece of forgetfulness to the MS. To avoid possible uncertainties, concerns or perhaps even recriminations, you should seek an objective assessment of any cognitive problems, if possible with a referral to a clinical psychologist, or more specifically to a neuropsychologist – usually from your neurologist.

Professional opinions

Until the results of recent research, many GPs and neurologists did not consider cognitive symptoms to be a major issue in relation to MS. Because the understanding and use of language is quite good in people with MS, in a single or occasional interview or consultation, it may be hard for a doctor to pick up more subtle but still important cognitive problems. As we have suggested, it is far more likely that those who are with you, and see you everyday, will notice these things first. People with MS have found that cognitive problems can be one of the main reasons why they have to go into residential care or why they become unemployed.

Tests

Formally, the range and extent of any cognitive problems can be measured and monitored through what are known as 'neuropsychological tests', usually given by a psychologist. They would involve some verbal and written tests focusing on things like your memory and your ability to solve problems of various kinds. These tests are becoming more sophisticated and you may be given a group (often called a 'battery') of tests that could take perhaps an hour or more to do. Your performance on these tests is then compared to those of normal healthy adults, and it is assumed that, unless there are other explanations, a much lower performance on one or more tests is due to MS. These tests are only given routinely in some clinical centres at present and, because this is still one of the developing areas of research and clinical practice in MS, you may need to attend specialist centres to obtain such an assessment.

Because some medications may affect your performance in tests, you should make the person who is testing you aware of what medication you are currently taking. The testing process itself may be problematic for other reasons. For example, many of the tests used for people with MS require a degree of coordination and manual dexterity, and this may be compromised by other effects of MS. Also, a problem in one area of cognition can affect performance in a test in an unrelated area, or it may be difficult to compare tests involving spoken responses with tests involving written or manual responses.

What might affect cognition?

Emotional state

Your emotional state may affect your cognitive performance, but the exact relationship and mechanism is not yet clear. Some studies have shown that depression seems to be related to cognitive performance, and others have shown the opposite.

Heat

Heat, or getting hot, may affect your cognitive performance, as it may influence other symptoms from time to time. Although little research has been undertaken on heat and cognition, on the basis of research on other symptoms it would be reasonable to conclude that if, for example, your memory could have been affected in this way, it would be likely to return to normal with a reduction in the temperature.

Medication

Medication may also affect cognition, particularly those that have central nervous system effects, such as sedatives, tranquillizers, certain pain killers and some steroid treatments. You should be aware of this possibility while you are doing everyday tasks that require concentration.

Cognitive problems found in MS

We must re-emphasise that the variability of cognitive problems in MS is very wide, some people do not have any cognitive problems and in others they are very mild. However, for information, the sort of problems that research has revealed are as follows. Memory loss is the most frequently found cognitive problem in MS. This may involve problems with short-term memory – failing to remember meetings or appointments, forgetting where things are and so on. There is also some evidence that people with MS may find it harder to learn new information. There are also difficulties with what is called abstract reasoning in some people with MS – that is the capacity to work with ideas and undertake analysis or decision-making in relation to such ideas. Sometimes speed of information processing may be affected in MS – things seem to take longer to think about and do. It may be more difficult to find words, and concentration can tend to wander more readily. In addition it is possible that capacity to organize things spatially becomes more difficult – for example putting together self-assembly furniture is more of a problem.

Management

Drugs

At present there are no drugs approved and accepted for the management of such problems as memory or concentration in MS. Memory problems are, of course, not limited to people with MS, and there is considerable research in this area. However, the cause of memory problems varies between different conditions, so drugs that might be helpful for people with Alzheimer's disease, who have very severe memory problems, would not necessarily be useful for people with MS. Nevertheless, there is increasing research to see whether a number of drugs, often originally developed for other purposes, might help people with MS.

There is some evidence that drugs used to assist fatigue may have modest effects on some cognitive problems. There are currently trials to see whether the drug pemoline might help cognitive function, and preliminary research on amantadine has suggested that it might have some effect on information processing. A drug with the proprietary name of Aricept, used for the treatment of memory disorders in Alzheimer's disease, is being studied to see whether it has any similar effects in people with MS. However, whilst in Alzheimer's disease this drug appears to increase the availability of a substance called acetylcholine, a neurotransmitter, this does not seem to be relevant to the cognitive problems in MS.

It is possible that beta-interferons and other recent drugs used to help manage MS itself may have some effect on cognitive function, for, as we have noted, that function tends to be more problematic the larger the number of lesions in the CNS. If the speed with which this increase is lessened, then there could be some effect on cognitive function. However, until recently, it has not been usual to include neuropsychological tests in clinical trials of such drugs, so further detailed research is needed and is now being undertaken.

Finally there has been publicity recently about the possible use of preparations of ginkgo biloba (made from the leaves of the *Ginkgo biloba* tree which grows in the Far East) for problems of memory and concentration. Trials of ginkgo biloba in people without MS have produced mixed results, early trials being promising but a major recent trial suggesting that it has little or no effect on memory and concentration. There have been no systematic trials on people with MS as yet and so no formal evidence that it could assist with their cognitive problems. In any case there are always problems in ensuring the purity of the active ingredient in such a product, and you should be cautious about its use.

Overall the investigation of possible drug therapies for cognitive problems is a large area of current research and it is hoped that major advances will be made in the next few years in this area.

Professional help

This is a very rapidly developing area of professional interest in relation to cognitive problems. Until recently, the main professions in these aspects of everyday living have been occupational and speech therapy. So, as part of the process of managing everyday activities, **occupational therapy** helps you to organize your environment, as well as your skills, to the maximum advantage. **Speech therapy** helps you with speech production problems, particularly if you take some time to articulate what you wish to say.

Some occupational therapists, particularly in North America and now in Britain, are developing special skills to help people with their memory and cognitive problems – often described collectively as **cognitive rehabilitation**. This is an approach designed to try and improve the everyday functioning of people with cognitive impairments resulting not only from MS but also other central nervous system disorders, such as head injury or stroke.

There are two broad approaches to cognitive rehabilitation. The first of these is to try to restore the lost functions, often through retraining, with the use of repetitive techniques such as learning lists, and helping people to re-acquire skills with progressively more complex tasks. The second is based on the idea that, because it will be difficult to regain the lost functions, compensatory strategies are needed, in which other devices and procedures are used, such as trying to minimize distractions, or using other means of reminding you about activities that you need to do. Both of these approaches are designed to help people manage their everyday lives better despite any cognitive impairment.

We need to repeat that cognitive rehabilitation, as a formal programme, is not available everywhere for people with MS. At present, following assessments, you will probably have most contact with an occupational therapist, whose skills focus substantially on the abilities needed to accomplish everyday activities, but we expect that many such therapists will increasingly be using at least some of the key techniques for managing problems that you may have in the area of memory or concentration.

Self-help

People with MS can be affected by a range of cognitive problems, and it is difficult to advise you precisely without knowing exactly what they are.

The difficulties often mentioned specifically – concentration and memory – are quite common.

Concentration. Everyone has occasional problems concentrating on things. Sometimes the problem is that we have many things going on at the same time – television, other people talking and a whole range of other activities going on. However, for someone with MS, concentrating on one of these activities – a conversation, for example – can be quite difficult, when so much else is happening. So the key thing is to try and have only one thing going on at a time – a conversation or the television, not both at the same time. You might have to move between rooms to achieve this. Find out when and where problems for you are most difficult, and then work on reducing the distractions to the minimum. Obviously changing your pattern of normal activities to help you concentrate may not be easy, but may be preferable to having continuing concentration problems.

Memory. There are many ways in which you can jog your memory. Some of these are routine, and may appear overpedantic or fussy for someone who has only minor memory difficulties, but all help to deal with short-term memory problems. For example, just making sure that clocks and watches show the right time; ensuring that today's date is prominently displayed somewhere; having a message board to note activities for today and tomorrow; having a list of activities that you are intending to do, with times and dates, perhaps in the form of a diary or similar record. Although this might seem almost too formal, note things down that you have agreed to do, or that you and others think important, so that it doesn't appear that you have forgotten it.

If you have difficulty with reading, check with your doctor whether you have any of the several potential eye problems associated with MS, that may interfere with your ability to read. Secondly, try and find a strategy to read in a particular way to maximize your ability to retain a story line.

As a broad guideline, the more of your senses that you use, the more likely you are to remember and retain ideas. Most people read things silently. It may be worth repeating what you read out loud, or at least key parts of it; or relate some elements of the story to another person; or write key ideas down. In this way, using more than one of your senses – writing, seeing, hearing and saying – you stand a better chance of remembering the story, or indeed other material. Admittedly, this approach may require some tolerant support from those around you but, if you are making a big effort to improve your memory, they will probably feel that they are gaining too.

You may find that you do not need to go to these lengths to help your memory – you could work out the main lines of the story or newspaper article by 'skim reading' so that, although you may have lost the element of surprise (about the ending of a story, for example!), you will have got an overall view of the text.

Depression

The incidence of depression amongst people with MS has been a matter of controversy for many years. In the early years of research it was thought that relatively few people with the condition had 'clinical' depression, but more recent research indicates that the level of depression is far higher than was previously thought.

Recent research suggests that up to 50% of people with MS (compared to only 5–15% of people without) will experience serious depression at some point in their lives, and at any one time perhaps one in seven may be experiencing this kind of depression. It is a very broad subject and could fill a book in its own right. An inspirational personal account on coping in MS is given in *Multiple Sclerosis – a personal exploration* by Dr Sandy Burnfield (see Appendix 2 for details).

Sometimes people ask about the incidence of suicide amongst people with MS. Although it is difficult to give precise figures, it does appear that the rate of suicide is higher for people with MS compared with the general population. There may be many reasons for this:

- Depression is associated with a higher rate of suicide – and as we have indicated people with MS have a higher rate of depression.
- There are also many other life crisis-based circumstances that may be linked with suicide whether or not people have MS.
- The consequences of having MS may, however, be linked more with things like general stress, employment problems, and problems with money, family or relationships, than for some other people.
- Also, when people feel a lack of hope for the future, sometimes suicide may seem an option.

In all these circumstances, it is very important that all avenues are explored for help, for through the management of depression and feelings of hopelessness, often situations that seem hopeless at the time are then viewed differently. Psychotherapy and or medication can assist greatly here.

Of course there is a related major debate under way, which is about the extent to which people can, or should be able to end their life if they wish – if necessary with assistance – if they are acting rationally knowing what they are doing and in full command of all their faculties. Such assistance is currently illegal in Great Britain and a number of recent high profile court cases have confirmed this position. This debate raises considerable emotions on all sides and no doubt will continue to be a matter of great controversy.

Management

As far as depression is concerned, it is important that you seek medical help partly because there are various forms of depression that may require different kinds of management. It is good that you have recognized that you may need help, because much can be done for you. Initially you may feel that seeking such help is a 'waste of time', or indeed carries with it some kind of stigma, similar to what people sometimes feel is associated with mental illness or 'weakness', but a sensible approach can substantially prevent you feeling miserable and improve your relationships.

Counselling and cognitive behaviour therapy

Depending on the nature of the depression, you may be offered counselling – and this is increasingly available both in general and hospital practice – or, rather more rarely, psychotherapy in larger and more specialist centres. In certain situations, where it may be helpful to discuss the depression in a family context, family therapy might be offered, although this again is very likely to be at the largest and most specialist centres. It is possible that these more specialist forms of therapy will involve onward referral, for assessment through a psychiatrist, for example. Cognitive behaviour therapy has been found very effective in some people with MS.

Drugs

More usually, you may be prescribed one of the antidepressant medications. Until recently, 'tricyclic antidepressants' were the most commonly used drugs, such as imipramine (Tofranil), amitryptiline (Elavil) and nortriptyline (Pamelor). However, another family of antidepressants, called 'serotinergic antidepressants', is now being prescribed much more regularly, drugs such as fluoxetine (Prozac), for example. These drugs have to be carefully administered and monitored, so it is important to follow medical advice. A combination of counselling **and** drug therapy may be needed.

Mood swings and euphoria

As far as emotional and attitudinal issues in MS are concerned, early research suggested that some people were emotionally labile (meaning their emotions fluctuated rapidly), and that other variable emotional symptoms or states arose that appeared to be specific to people with the disease. However, it proved difficult to tell whether the problems were a personal – indeed an emotional – reaction to the onset of MS, or were caused by the MS itself. Current research is indicating that there are problems of an emotional kind that might be linked to the disease itself, as well as personal reactions to it.

Mood swings may be caused by the effects of demyelination in particular parts of the central nervous system that control moods and emotions, or by everyday frustrations and issues that arise in managing and thinking about the effects of MS. Either way, recognizing that mood swings exist is the first step in being able to manage them more effectively.

In more extreme cases, mood swings are referred to medically as a 'bipolar disorder', with relatively rapid and severe swings between depression and elation. Medical assistance should be sought in such cases.

Euphoria

One of the first symptoms that doctors described over 150 years ago was an 'elevation of mood' in some people with MS. This was also called 'an unusual cheerfulness' that seemed not quite appropriate in someone with a long-term medical condition. In fact, some of these attributions of 'elevated mood' were not linked to the MS itself, but to the circumstances in which it was diagnosed. However, since that time, the idea that some people with MS may occasionally have what is often described as 'euphoria' has become more accepted. This can be linked with mood swings that may take people with MS through a range of emotions from depression, perhaps to anger and indeed to 'euphoria' over a period of time.

The previous clinical concern with euphoria has led to far less attention being paid to the much more serious problem of depression, which we have just discussed. It is possible that, in some people with MS, a euphoric presentation has cloaked an underlying depression. Euphoria is viewed as a widespread phenomenon because of the very positive reactions – the relief almost – that some people with MS feel once diagnosed. Because the process, and the communication more so, of the diagnosis may take some time, some people felt that their symptoms may have been due to even more serious conditions – a brain tumour, for example, or that they were 'going mad'. Some doctors have treated the, often profound, relief of some of their patients on hearing that they 'only' have MS, as indicating a euphoric state caused by the MS, rather than an understandable relief that they have a condition far less threatening than others they had feared.

Although inappropriate laughter may occasionally be embarrassing, it seems to be a result of damage to a particular part of the nervous system, and may require professional help to manage – this particular phenomenon of 'euphoria' seems to be overemphasized and, in terms of everyday symptom management, other emotional problems, particularly those centred around depression, are more harmful and significant.

Effects of drugs

Any drug that has powerful effects on symptoms is likely to have a wider range of effects – what we usually call 'side effects' – that we don't usually want. In particular, drugs that act in various ways on symptoms related to the central nervous system may well have effects on your moods and feelings.

Steroid drugs in particular – still quite widely used in relation to managing attacks or exacerbations of MS – may have mood-changing properties. These properties are not always predictable, and people can sometimes have quite strong reactions to steroid drugs. Perversely, some people may feel more depressed, while others may feel more cheerful on them. There is something which has become known as a steroid 'high', where people can become more active (indeed 'hyperactive') on the drugs, and then feel a 'low' when they come off them; others may experience quite bad mood changes from such drugs. Try monitoring yourself and get a family member to discuss any changes that they see in you, and then report such changes to your neurologist or other doctor treating you.

Some other drugs may have mood-changing effects, especially if you suddenly increase or decrease the dose that you are taking. For example, baclofen (Lioresal), a drug very widely used to control spasticity, has been known to produce major effects on mood; for example, if a high dose is withdrawn suddenly, people may feel very agitated, experience substantial mood changes, or even hallucinate. So is sensible to report any untoward reactions that you may have with your drugs to your GP or neurologist before gradually reducing the dosage. Other drugs, such as diazepam (Valium), used for relaxing muscles, may make you feel very relaxed! Sometimes low doses of antidepressants, used to treat urinary problems or some sensory symptoms, may also change your mood.

Although we don't want to exaggerate the number of mood or emotional reactions that you might have to the drugs being taken for symptoms, these additional side effects, which can occur relatively soon after you have decreased or increased doses, may be caused by them. If you are in doubt, report your symptoms to your GP or neurologist, and seek their advice as to how best to manage them.

Management of mood swings

Family and friends are often the first people to recognize that mood swings are occurring. For all of us, relationships with other people are bound up with knowing what they will do in a relatively predictable way. If this expectation breaks down, as it may do if mood swings (technically described as 'emotional lability') are serious, then family relationships may suffer substantially. For some families these problems can be very difficult to handle, and thus external advice and help can be sought.

Counselling and/or drugs and cognitive behaviour therapy

After a consultation with your GP or neurologist, you may be able to get counselling or have a systematic discussion of your family and personal problems arising from the mood swings; if counselling fails, a tricyclic antidepressant (such as amitriptyline) might be prescribed. There is also increasing but still unsystematic evidence that fluoxetine (Prozac) may offer some help in this situation. As we noted earlier, previous administrations of steroids – usually to treat exacerbations of the MS – may have prompted some increase in mood swings (see above), in which case a drug such as lithium or carbamazepine might reduce these swings. Cognitive behaviour therapy has been found useful also in people with mood swings in MS.

Self-help

Often your emotional response to a situation may be just rather 'too strong' for the particular situation concerned. You could try breathing deeply, pausing before the tears or laughter come, particularly in stressful situations. If you find yourself laughing or crying without any apparent cause – indeed your mood may be totally at variance with this expression of emotion – and it is difficult to stop, almost certainly this is a result of damage caused by MS itself, probably to areas of the brain controlling the release of emotional expression. This problem has to be managed socially, which is not an easy task, but you could be prescribed medications which have some dampening effect on the release of emotions. It would be best to consult your GP or neurologist about these matters.

8

Mobility and managing everyday life

Mobility or movement problems can be variable depending on the overall disease development, and on whether you are currently in the middle of an attack or in remission. The main aim is to maintain as much mobility as possible, in particular to avoid what might be called 'secondary' damage in the form of wasting ('atrophied') muscles, which occurs as a result of prolonged lack of use.

In the early stages of MS, movement problems may be relatively limited or infrequent, and indeed many people find that they can continue physically with almost all the things that they did before. You may have sometimes to temper or reduce the more vigorous of your activities. As long as you are relatively active, are sensible in relation to the overall approach to exercise, and do not appear to have significant individual problems of movement, you may not need professional help or support at this stage. Do talk the situation over with your neurologist or, failing that, your GP, both of whom can refer you to professional help if they feel it necessary. Sometimes movement problems can creep up on you and, without realizing it (or perhaps not wanting to realize it), you may need more help than you first thought. In general, exercise is best thought of as a preventative process, not so much a curative one, so it is best undertaken at an early stage.

Professional help

Although there has been an explosion of health and fitness clubs, which might be thought to help people with mobility or other similar difficulties, very few of them have staff who will be aware of MS and its effects on movement. So it's a good idea to seek the help of members of the key profession dealing with mobility and movement problems, and that is physiotherapy. Normally you will be referred for a consultation with a physiotherapist by your neurologist or GP. Check, either with your referring doctor or with the physiotherapist, that they have had experience of managing people with MS.

A physiotherapist will normally undertake a number of assessments of your movement ability. These would include generally:

- evaluating your general posture and body movements;
- taking account not only of what you can do in the clinic, surgery or hospital, but also what problems you may have in and around the home and work;
- measuring the strength of various muscles, as well as assessing how flexible your joints, tendons and muscles are;
- testing the sensations that you may have in or around your muscles, as well as your ability to sense cold and heat.

Some physiotherapists, particularly in leading hospitals, may undertake what is called 'gait analysis', i.e. a formal assessment of how you move, particularly how you walk, investigating things like speed, rhythm of movement, stride and step length. This analysis helps to determine exactly where your movement problems lie in order to help correct them. Physiotherapists increasingly like to know about your own history and your worries about your movement problems, and to try and work with them, as well as with those problems that they have detected themselves.

Exercises

A physiotherapist would normally recommend a programme of management geared to the diagnosis of your mobility problems.

The main aim of exercising is to:

- try and keep as many muscles as possible in good working order;
- strengthen those that have become weak;
- help keep joints mobile;
- help prevent them from getting stiff;
- help your coordination and balance;
- improve your circulation – and in doing so help other body functions;
- help reduce spasticity in more advanced MS;
- help prevent pressure sores.

Types of exercise

A number of different types of exercise might be recommended depending on this diagnosis.

- For your overall fitness, **general exercises** may be recommended, not necessarily linked to any particular movement symptom of your MS.
- **Exercises to improve your *cardiovascular* fitness** will increase your heart rate, and are good for your circulation.
- **Stretching exercises** will decrease the risk of spasticity and contractures. These exercises work by stretching muscles and tendons to increase their flexibility and elasticity.
- **Resistance exercises**, with the use of weights or other devices, help increase the strength of muscles that have been weakened.
- **Range of motion exercises** focus on improving the degree of motion of joints in the body, and aim to overcome, as far as possible, difficulties caused by stiffness in joints or problems in tendons and ligaments.

There are several different ways in which exercises may be undertaken:

- What are called **active exercises** are those that you can undertake yourself without any help, and you may use weights or changes of position to give more resistance (to increase the value of the exercise).
- **Self-assisted exercises** are ones in which you can use one part of your body to assist another, e.g. by using a stronger arm to assist a weaker arm.
- **Active assisted exercises** are those in which another person is needed to help you from time to time, but in which you still do most of the exercising yourself.
- **Passive exercises** are those performed on you by others when you cannot easily move yourself, e.g. moving your arms or legs for you, to increase the range of motion.

As you can see from these different types of exercise, you will not always need to have the physiotherapist present. Even in relation to passive or active assisted exercises, other people, once they know how to help, can assist you. Indeed the normal pattern is for you to have an assessment and a small number of sessions with a physiotherapist initially – usually five or six over a period of a few weeks – and then for you to work on the agreed exercises on your own or with a member of your family. You would probably return to the physiotherapist for periodic assessments thereafter to check how you are getting on.

Self-help exercises

Overall, one could say that exercise will help you maintain your maximum independence. Some floor and chair exercises are shown in Figures 8.1 and 8.2. Passive exercise is shown in Figure 8.3.

Regular sessions

Many people with MS find it puzzling, or even very disturbing, that physiotherapists will see them and assist them directly for several sessions, and then end regular consultations. This is for the following reasons:

- Pressures of time and resources mean that it is difficult for physiotherapists to continue to give regular (weekly or fortnightly) sessions beyond the initial phase of therapy.
- The training of physiotherapists emphasizes their evaluating role, in which the onus is on transferring responsibility as much as possible to the patient (client) for continuation of an agreed exercise programme.

An important feature of exercise is that it continues on a regular basis and that as much as possible is undertaken by the person with MS. Unfortunately, there is often a conflict between the view of physiotherapists, who consider that one of their main tasks is to ensure that people with MS undertake an agreed programme on their own or with family assistance, and the views of people with MS, who often feel that the support provided by regular and continuing visits to a physiotherapist is vital. It is often difficult to resolve this conflict, although some pattern of occasional consultations can often be agreed.

Caution

Be careful not to get overheated or exhausted, which may on occasion lead to a temporary increase in some MS symptoms (see Chapter 6). Your own commonsense will normally tell you when you are exerting yourself too much. Generally, if you exercise carefully and regularly, with periodic breaks, you should find that you can get the most reward from the exercise.

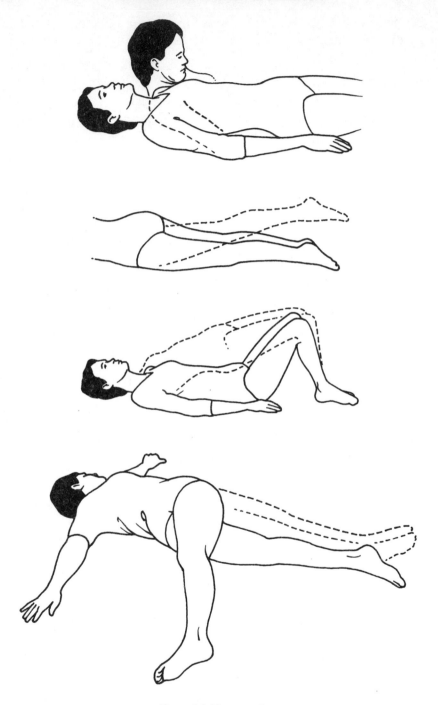

Figure 8.1 Floor exercises.

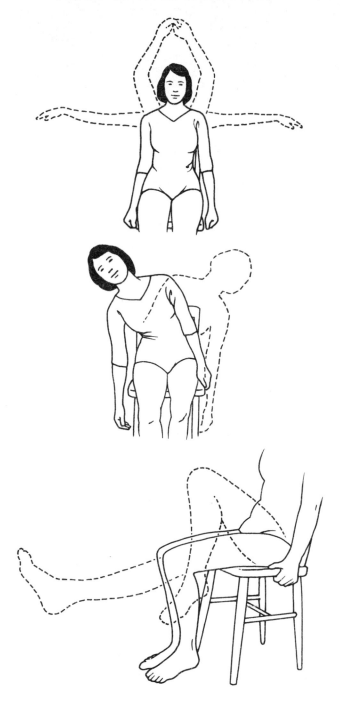

Figure 8.2 Chair exercises.

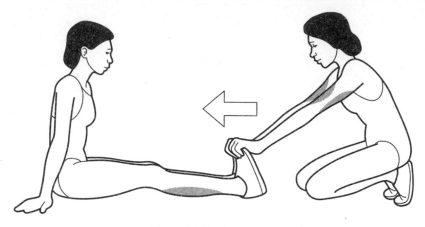

Figure 8.3 Passive exercise.

Having a helper

In general, the physiotherapist should have indicated how a friend or partner can help but, apart from following those instructions carefully, the following broad points may apply:

- Get them to encourage you to undertake as much movement as possible, but don't let them impede your movements.
- They should allow you to perform a passive exercise (an exercise undertaken with/on a person by another person), as smoothly as possible.
- They shouldn't apply increased pressure at the most extreme points of the movement and, if a spasm occurs when they touch a limb, wait to see whether the spasm ceases and then let them help for as long as the movement is comfortable.

Guidelines

Most of the guidelines are quite sensible if you think about them.

- Try and undertake those exercises that you have been recommended to do by a physiotherapist regularly, preferably every day – unless the physiotherapist indicates otherwise.
- Whether you have been given advice by a physiotherapist or not, it would be wise to try and move around as much as you can, and to sit and stand as erect as possible. Posture is very important. When

it is bad, it may produce muscle and joint strains, and secondary back problems. Furthermore, bad posture in a wheelchair or other chair may have more profound constrictive effects on your breathing and chest.

- Try to exercise within your own capacity, i.e. do not get overtired, and try not to worry if you perform less well on a bad day. Everybody's performance varies from day to day.
- Also try and recognize when you need professional advice about problems that you are experiencing and that are not being helped by your current pattern of exercises.

Sports

The diagnosis of MS in itself should make no difference as to whether you continue to play sports or not. The key issues are whether you enjoy playing the sport, whether you feel that you can play the sport as well, or nearly as well, as you did before, and whether you feel that there are any inherent problems, e.g. a significant risk of injury, that might affect your life in other ways. People without MS have to consider these issues as well. You might be able to change your approach to sport later, perhaps by playing at a different level, if you feel that there may be problems for you at the highest competitive level. Nevertheless, sporting exercise is good for you, especially if you enjoy and benefit from it.

Fatigue and exercises

If you feel too tired to exercise, the key to solving this problem may be working out ways in which you can take advantage of the times when you feel less fatigued in order to do modest but well-targeted exercise. Look carefully at the day-to-day activities you undertake, to see whether they might be rearranged and result in less fatigue. Sometimes, introducing rest periods and using specific aids for certain activities will result in less fatigue, and the chance to undertake limited and helpful exercises. You may also need, perhaps in consultation with a physiotherapist, to review the exercises to make them less vigorous. After all, it is not only a question of getting your exercise regimen right, but of getting a good balance between exercise and relaxation.

Weakness and exercise

Physiotherapy, or exercise in general, cannot 'mend' the damaged nerve fibres that lead to less effective control of muscles. Weakness in the legs, and problems of balance, may be due directly to less effective nerve conduction, but exercise may help other causes of weakness. Devise a programme of exercise with your physiotherapist making sure that any special exercises that you do undertake, e.g. resistance exercises through using weights, are in fact likely to help you.

After an MS attack, some people find that they cannot walk. Whilst normally some recovery is usual from the symptoms experienced at the height of an attack, the extent of this recovery can vary a lot. If demyelination has been quite substantial, there is little you can do through an exercise programme to reduce this damage, but you should still do leg exercises in order to keep your muscles as strong as possible, and to maintain flexibility so that, if more spontaneous recovery occurs, you will be able to take advantage of this. In any case it is very important to continue undertaking leg exercises, so that you can sit more comfortably and avoid some of the problems that can come with prolonged sitting.

Spasticity and exercise

A regular programme of stretching and related exercises can help muscular development, or at the very least help prevent the muscles wasting away. Keep your joints, tendons and ligaments as flexible as possible. Avoid positions where spasticity is more likely. Keep your head as central as possible when doing exercises and, if spasticity does occur, do a passive exercise as smoothly as possible to relax your muscles. On occasion it has been found that towels dipped in iced water and applied to the relevant area for a few minutes at most may help the muscles to relax. Unfortunately, as MS progresses, even with the most helpful exercise programme, additional means – usually prescribed drugs – may be necessary to assist the spasticity. You should consult your neurologist or GP about these.

Swimming

Swimming is a good form of exercise for everyone, but especially for people with MS, because your body weight is supported by the water. Weakened muscles can operate in this environment and will strengthen from the resistance. In addition, as swimming involves many muscle systems in your body, it can help to increase coordination.

Your main practical problems may be issues such as where the changing rooms are in relation to the pool, and obtaining assistance to reach, and return from, the pool. There are now more and more swimming pools and leisure centres offering special sessions for people who need special help, and it might be worth trying one of these sessions at first. If such sessions are not available, try lobbying your local leisure centre/swimming pool for one. It may be worth asking whether there are quiet times of the day when the pool will be freer, and assistance is more likely to be available.

Functional electrical stimulation (FES) can help some people with 'foot drop'. A small box sends electrical stimulation to muscles in the lower leg, so that you can regain useful movement. This is connected to a pressure pad in a shoe that enables the impulse to be triggered when you are walking, improving mobility. (See Appendix 1 for address of the FES Team.)

One point may prove to be important and that is the temperature of the water. The temperature that many people with MS find comfortable is about 30°C (86°F). Much lower temperatures appear to be too cold, although still tolerable, whereas much higher temperatures, often found in jacuzzis or spa baths, are sometimes associated with the onset of (temporary) MS symptoms. Also, in relation to your swimming activities, if you have troublesome bladder control, it may be worth discussing this with your neurologist or GP beforehand to try and ease your concerns.

Foot drop and exercise

'Foot drop' occurs when the muscles of the foot and ankle become weak, caused by poor nerve conduction, and either your ankle may just 'turn over' or, more commonly, your toes touch the ground before your heel – in contrast to the normal heel–toe action – and this might lead you to fall. This is quite a common problem in MS. There are two ways of dealing with it. One way is by exercising the relevant muscles as much as possible, through passive exercises if necessary. However, this may not be enough to prevent the problem once it has occurred. A special brace may be helpful, which supports the weakened ankle and allows you to walk again with the normal heel and toe action, if your leg muscles are strong enough to allow this (Figure 8.4). You may need to consider using a wheelchair or scooter, at least occasionally.

One of your feet 'turning in' is another problem that some people with MS have. In this situation the muscles turning the foot out have weakened, and the muscles and tendons on the inside of the foot have become shortened – largely due to disuse. In addition the ankle joint may be more rigid and stiff. Thus it is vital for people with MS to try and prevent such a situation occurring by exercising the muscles controlling the ankle as much as possible. It will be important to seek some help from a

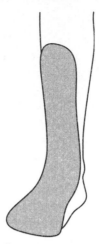

Figure 8.4 Leg brace.

physiotherapist when the problem has arisen to ensure that you undertake the correct exercises and, if necessary, have a supporting brace.

Wheelchairs and exercise

Although it may sound paradoxical, it is almost more important for someone confined to a wheelchair to undertake regular exercise than someone who can walk. You should try and undertake exercises that maintain the movement and flexibility in your joints as much as possible – through the 'range of motion' and stretching exercises described earlier. As far as possible, try and maintain also your upper body strength – this is particularly important for good posture, which itself will help prevent some of the more problematic aspects of being in a wheelchair for a long time. Exercising your neck muscles will also help you to maintain a good posture. If possible, it is very helpful just to stand for a few minutes each day, with the help of someone else or with an increasing range of equipment now available for this purpose. It is known that bone density tends to decrease (causing 'osteoporosis') more quickly if weight is not borne by the legs and feet on a regular basis and low bone density is also one of the contributory factors of fractures. This is another reason why standing should, if possible, be undertaken – even if only for a very short period. As with sitting in a chair, you ought to learn specific exercises to be able to shift your weight on a regular basis, to prevent skin breakdown at the points where your body is in contact with the wheelchair, and ultimately to prevent pressure sores. (See Figure 8.2 for exercises that you can do sitting down.)

Pressure sores

As noted earlier, exercise can help prevent pressure sores. They are very dangerous once they arise, and yet they are entirely preventable. Basically, as the name suggests, they arise when the skin begins to break down from too much continuous pressure, from a chair or bed, for example, on key points of your body. Once this pressure has been applied for a long time, blood circulation to the area lessens or ceases, the tissues get starved of oxygen, and the skin and related tissues break down. Such pressure sores are particularly dangerous because, left untreated, they can lead to infection of the underlying bare tissue or to blood infection ('septicaemia'), which can threaten your life. Most people do not get pressure sores because they move very frequently and thus pressure is never exerted on one point of their body for long enough for a pressure

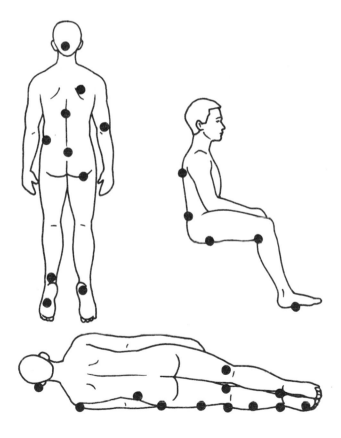

Figure 8.5 Pressure sore areas.

sore to develop. Danger areas are the lower back, the shoulder blades, the insides of knees, hips, elbows, ankles, heels, toes, wrists, and even sometimes ears (Figure 8.5). Pressure sores are more likely if you are in a wheelchair, or are sitting or in bed for long periods of time.

Initially, a pressure sore may just look like an area of reddened skin, or even a small bruise. It can look like a blister or weal, which may break to reveal a small or even a large hole where the skin has been damaged more fundamentally. It is likely to be very painful but, if sensation has been lost, you may not be aware an ulcer is forming so visual checks are also necessary. It is important to act immediately and contact your doctor, for once the damage has occurred it is very unlikely to get better without considerable treatment.

Preventative therapy, i.e. regular movement every hour or two, is vital, especially for people in wheelchairs or in bed. If you can stand for even a short time, or shift your weight from time to time and from place to place, this is helpful. There are also a number of products that may help:

- ripple mattresses
- foam rings
- gel or air cushions
- water beds
- pads
- specific textures of clothing and bedding, especially sheepskin.

Sometimes the bedclothes can be lifted off the body by means of a cradle. You should wear nightdresses or pyjamas that chafe as little as possible.

The usual person to treat pressure sores is a District Nurse who will come in regularly to manage them. The treatment usually involves antibiotic cream or powder in and around the area. The aim is to prevent infection and to restore circulation, by keeping the skin clean and dry. The sore may be left exposed to the air during the day, but dressed with a sterile dressing at night. More serious sores may require substantial hospital treatment.

There is a great deal of development work currently underway on the management of pressure sores because, not only are they very painful, inconvenient and potentially dangerous for people with MS, but they are also very expensive to treat, at home or in hospital, and often involve very long-term nursing and medical care.

Aids and equipment

Occupational therapy

Many of the aids and much of the equipment that you might need are available through an occupational therapist or at least you are likely to be able to obtain their advice on what to have. Occupational therapy is mainly concerned with helping people to manage any difficulties they may have in 'daily living'. You will almost certainly be offered a consultation with an occupational therapist (OT) at some point but, if you are not and want such professional advice, your GP or neurologist should be able to refer you to an OT to assist you. You also may need to use an OT if you wish to obtain aids and equipment through your local NHS Trust or Department of Social Services.

Walking aids

Many people with MS experience problems in walking. Sometimes this is temporary, e.g. during an attack or exacerbation, sometimes it is more long term as the MS develops. A major problem is often a difficulty with balance, causing staggering, in which you fear you may fall. Of course, using a mobility aid (walking stick, crutch, and so on) is something that many people with MS dread, for it appears to be a very visible sign both to yourself and others that the MS is progressing. However, once your balance has started to deteriorate significantly, people with MS often report that, when others see them, with no mobility aid, staggering and losing their balance, they seem to think that the person with MS is drunk. Thus dealing with this problem is important socially and physically, to prevent falls and possible injury.

A mobility aid is the usual way to overcome these problems, and your physiotherapist or OT can help here. Mobility aids range from one or two canes (walking sticks), to one or two crutches used under the forearms, to light walkers which have four legs (Figure 8.6). Both canes and crutches can have several short legs to give increased stability. Ensure that whatever you use deals with the problems you have or might have, and that you are comfortable using it. You may need to experiment a bit to get the right combination of mobility aids for different situations. For example, although some people are worried that walkers are amongst the most visible of mobility aids, because they operate in front of you they give you more stability, and may even reduce fatigue from walking. They may also have a seat, or a basket to

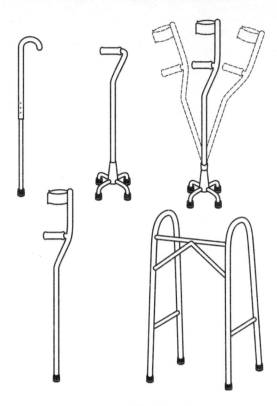

Figure 8.6 Mobility aids.

allow you to carry things. Keep your situation under review, and make sure that the mobility aid you are currently using is really the one best for you.

Chairs and wheelchairs

For many people with MS, the day when they feel that they have to consider using a wheelchair is a big day in their lives. However, we all have to adapt to declining mobility as we get older, and to using additional means of getting around. Although there is still some social stigma attached to being in a wheelchair, the situation has dramatically changed in the last few years: in particular, changes in wheelchair design, the use of wheelchairs for highly successful sports activities, and the advent of the electric scooter mean less dependence on others than previously.

Sometimes the use of a wheelchair may be a relief – in the sense that it can help avoid some of the most awkward and exhausting struggles to get around, both for you or your partner or family members. In any case, you may only need it on an occasional basis.

Guidelines for choosing a chair

The general rule is, of course, that you should choose a chair that is comfortable for you – particularly when you are using it for longer periods. However comfortable the chair, you must move regularly, at the very least by shifting your position, to try and avoid pressure sores and enhance your circulation. Maintaining a good posture is especially crucial if you are sitting for long periods. More specifically, the height of your chair should be such that your hips, knees and ankles rest at right angles. The depth should allow your thighs to be well supported without undue pressure behind the knee, and arm rests should be set at a height where your shoulders are relaxed when your forearms are placed on the rests. You should also have a chair that allows your head to be supported.

When to buy a wheelchair

It is best to make a gradual transition to wheelchair use, if you can, over weeks, months or years. When you find that:

- the effort, perhaps particularly outside the home, required to walk some distance is too much;
- walking aids tend to assist you less;
- you are getting increasingly concerned about falling

then it will be worth considering using a wheelchair, at least for some activities.

All but a few people with MS should be able to make a gradual transition to a wheelchair. This may overcome the 'all or nothing' approach, which many people with MS fear.

If it is outside the home that you need to use a wheelchair first, you could think of getting around in a combination of ways: using a wheelchair for some things and a walking aid for others. Where there are sufficient supports – perhaps around the home – you may be able to walk relatively unaided for a few steps. In this way, you can conserve your precious energy, still undertake some active exercise, and maybe actually increase the range of activities that you are able to do.

Advice

It is important that you obtain good independent advice about the appropriate type and specification of wheelchair for your needs. An increasing number of companies are now producing wheelchairs of all kinds but it is best to ask someone who professionally assesses wheelchairs, usually an occupational therapist or a physiotherapist. The NHS also operates Wheelchair Service Centres, where assessment is undertaken, and to which you should be referred for advice.

You might be able to get financial help via the mobility components of the Disability Living Allowance. See the section on *Benefits* in Chapter 13.

Types

There are several types of wheelchair that you need to consider depending on your circumstances (Figure 8.7):

- Up until recently the most common was a **manual wheelchair**, powered by yourself – for which you need sufficient upper body strength and, for going some distance, endurance, and relatively low and predictable levels of fatigue.
- For people who may need to use a wheelchair from time to time, **portable (collapsible) wheelchairs** are available to take with you in a car.
- **Powered wheelchairs** are increasingly used by someone who cannot stand well or transfer easily, and has not got sufficient upper body strength to propel a wheelchair manually. They are usually driven by means of a small control arm, battery driven, heavy and very solid, and are not easily transportable – so a specially adapted car or van into which the wheelchair can be driven is usually needed.
- A very popular, but relatively expensive, alternative for people who have not got the upper body strength to propel a manual wheel-chair, but who can stand, transfer well and have reasonable balance, is an **electric scooter**. The scooter looks like an electric golf cart – it is battery driven with three or four wheels, and is steered and controlled through the handlebars. There are now many types of electric scooter, some of them relatively portable, although they are still very heavy.

Powered wheelchairs, and particularly electric scooters, are enabling people with MS to have a radically new approach, not only to their mobility but also and just as important, to their social relationships. Rather than being pushed from behind, people now feel more in control. They can move at the pace of others, talk to them side by side and establish again a more equal – and independent – relationship, at least in this aspect of their lives. Research is now indicating how important the advent of electric scooters is for opening a new phase in the mobility of people with MS.

Which is best for you?

The criteria used to assess which type of mobility aid is best suited to you are generally:

- your ability to stand, balance and transfer;
- your ability to use the controls on a powered chair or vehicle;
- your upper body strength;
- the nature of your activities, particularly the balance between indoor and outdoor activities;
- the terrain outside and inside your house, and
- the availability of someone to assist you.

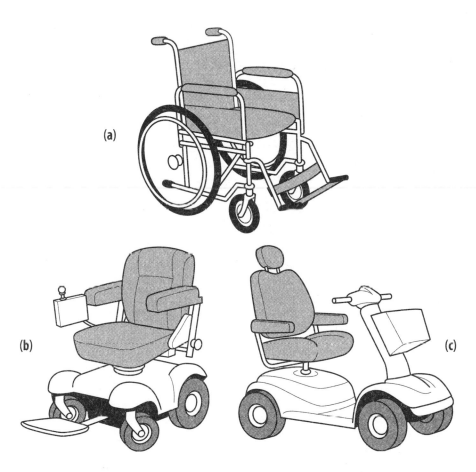

Figure 8.7 Wheelchair types: (**a**) manual, (**b**) powered, (**c**) electric scooter.

Your memory and cognitive status will be assessed if, for example, you are likely to travel very far on your own. Professional advisors like to reduce to the minimum any risks that you might run by using a vehicle such as a scooter – you may feel it is appropriate for you to have one, but they may feel that you are only just able to control it. This view frustrates people with MS who sometimes feel their capacities are greater than those estimated by their professional advisor.

Negotiating between wheelchair and chair

When your leg muscles are weak, and the neurological control of them is very damaged, moving from a seated to an upright position is often very difficult. You may well need some professional advice and demonstration as to how best to accomplish this – possibly with aids, or someone who can help. As a general rule be sure you have any walking aid that you regularly use nearby, wear shoes, and always stand on a non-slip surface. The usual procedure to get up is to put your feet slightly apart and flat on the floor, and then to pull them back a little towards the chair. Place both hands on the chair arms, and then ease yourself forward so that your bottom is near the front of the chair. Then lean slightly forward, lift your head and look straight in front. You should then push down on your hands and heels, and straighten your hips and knees.

When you move from a standing to a sitting position, the procedure is rather simpler, and involves turning round, so that you can feel the chair with the back of your legs. Use the chair arms to lower yourself into position. Of course, if you are getting in and out of a wheelchair, ensure that the chair is stable and that the wheelchair brakes are on! It is possible that in time you might need further assistance. There are inflatable and portable cushions to help you rise from a chair, and there are also a number of mechanical aids, usually incorporated into the chairs themselves, that hydraulically assist the actions of sitting and standing – although these can be expensive.

Bathroom aids

Baths and showers

Ensure that getting in and out of the bath is as safe and easy as possible and that, when you are in the bath, you can relax without worrying. Working out how to clean yourself properly is often a relatively minor problem compared to getting in and out of the bath! Negotiating a bath requires both balance and strength. There are several things that can be done in stages (Fig. 8.8):

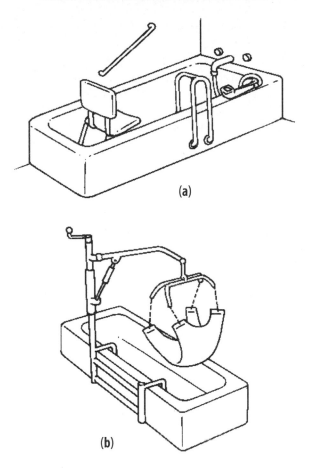

Figure 8.8 Bath aids: (**a**) grab bars and seat; (**b**) hoist.

- Ensure that non-slip mats are both in the bath and on the floor.
- Install grab bars at crucial points so that you can lower yourself in and pull yourself out. The siting of these is very important – consult your occupational therapist or other skilled person, to make sure that they can really help you.
- Even if there is not someone else actually in the bathroom with you, it is good to have someone you can call on if you do get into difficulty.
- If grab bars are not sufficient, perhaps because you have not got enough strength to use them, then you may need to consider other options, including bath seats both for transfer, and for use in the bath.

- Bath hoists are also available that help to lift you in and out of your bath.
- Another possibility, if it proves too difficult to negotiate the bath, is to install a shower: the larger types will have sufficient space for a shower chair or bench to sit on and will be easier to access than a bath. With a hand-held, temperature-controlled shower attachment, you should have a reasonably enjoyable experience, even if it isn't quite the same for some people as a bath!

Toilet aids

Toiletting aids are important for, traditionally in our society, going to the toilet yourself is an indication of independence. Continuing to go to the toilet completely by yourself for as long as possible is an issue that many people feel strongly about, even between partners who have known each other for many years. Although having other people to assist you is a problem for both sexes, many men in particular are not so used to helping others with such issues on an everyday basis, such as young children or older parents, or indeed their partners.

Clothing. A number of procedures can help. For men, one of the first things that you could do, if you have difficulties in controlling finger movement, is to readjust your type of clothing, to enable you to urinate from a standing position, or to take off or loosen your trousers and underwear. Buttons on trousers are not often not easy to manage, so a zip is usually slightly more user friendly; if zips are difficult to operate, Velcro fastenings will still look good and fasten well; they can be used on underwear as well. Women may find this similarly helpful when they are wearing trousers.

Toilet. If you have limited movement, or are a bit unsteady, you will need to be very careful in lowering yourself on to the toilet. You need to check where your arms and feet are, and stand directly in front of the seat, then bend your knees until you can touch the sides of the seat with your hands, and lower yourself down slowly. When raising yourself use the toilet seat to push yourself off. Check that the toilet seat is secure before embarking on lowering or raising yourself!

As far as the toilet itself is concerned, there are a range of adaptations which may be of help:

- Grab bars can be placed on adjacent walls if they are near enough.
- Where a toilet is standing away from a wall, you could consider an over-the-toilet adjustable frame, which has arm-rests to help you raise and lower yourself (Fig. 8.9).

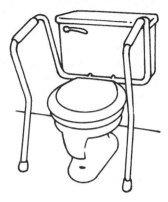

Figure 8.9 Over-the-toilet frame.

- There is an increasingly wide range of commodes.
- You can install a slightly elevated toilet seat.

The number of different adaptations in this area is increasing rapidly, so consult your occupational therapist, and look at other sources of information about such products.

Toilet paper. One of the most trying problems for people with MS is using toilet paper, for the manoeuvre involves considerable movement and dexterity. You might find a wet cloth more useful than toilet paper, or you might consider using a squeezy bottle full of (warm!) water. There is also special equipment, such as a toilet-paper holder, which could help. A bidet might be easier, although this may well not fit into your toilet area, can be rather expensive to install, and would need fitting to your water supply. Recently a portable toilet/bidet has been launched that might help people who are worried about travelling and having to deal with conventional, and therefore problematic, toilets elsewhere. You may find a toilet that automatically washes and dries you where you are – this is the kind of development that could help many people with MS considerably.

Public toilets. Finally, when you are out and about, you can obtain a special key from RADAR for public toilets for disabled people. More and more of these toilets are being made available.

Dressing aids

The problem with dressing, or undressing for that matter, if you have limited movement and dexterity, is not just the difficulty but also the time involved in doing them. Although you may be able to accomplish dressing now, in due course it can become such a frustrating and time-consuming process, that you have got little energy left to do anything else. As usual, it is a compromise between attempting to use all the traditional fittings on clothing, and having some which are easier to do up or undo. Of course everyone wants to look good in the clothes they are wearing, and it is often a question of trying to balance being fashionable (or not being unfashionable!) with clothes that are easy to manage. Women are in a slightly better position socially than men, in being able to use more accessories, such as jewellery or scarves, to complement whatever clothes they are wearing.

In general, tight-fitting clothes are harder to manage than looser ones, whatever kinds of fixings are on them. Try:

- large rather than small buttons;
- trousers or skirts with elasticated waists;
- dressing aids such as dressing sticks and button hooks.

One of the trickiest problems for men is that of collars, ties and buttoned shirts. Most of the buttons on shirts can be left done up, so that the shirts can be slipped over the head, If this is a problem, buttonholes can be closed, then the buttons sewn on the outside of the shirt and Velcro strips placed behind them, so that when all the strips are closed it looks as though the shirt is buttoned in the traditional way. As far as ties are concerned, clip-on ones may be easier to use than the usual hand-tied ones or, alternatively, ties can be left already loosely tied and slipped over the head, and then tightened in place.

Shoes and socks

These cause real problems for people with MS, for they involve a range of movement, together with fine dexterity, both of which can be compromised. One way forward is to investigate the possibility of different ways of tying your shoes. If you are able to reach your shoes, then there are Velcro shoe fastenings, and various devices to tighten laces, and you can learn single-handed tying techniques. If you cannot reach your shoes, then slip-on shoes are a better idea; you could convert your lace-up shoes into slip-ons with elastic laces, if the shoe tongue can be stitched into place. Long-handled shoe horns will help you put on slip-on shoes.

There are a range of other aids available to help pull on (and take off) socks and tights – these usually work through gripping the socks or tights with the end of a hand-operated long-handled tool.

Bed aids

People with MS often find it hard not so much getting into the bed but getting out of it again, in particular, getting up from low, and particularly soft, mattresses.

You can try rolling onto your side and, facing the edge of the bed, try pushing yourself up with your underneath arm and, at the same time, swinging your legs over the bed. Once you are sitting up with your legs on the ground, it becomes easier to push up from the bed. There are some other things that you could try:

- Cloth strips attached to the mattress will help you to pull yourself up.
- You could position a grab bar, or even a floor-to-ceiling bar nearby, so that you can manoeuvre yourself to a standing position.
- A bedpull (a rope or piece of strong webbing) lying on top of the bed and attached to the floor or other secure object, or a frame resting by the side of the bed could help.
- You can raise the bed, but do ensure that this is done securely.

If these strategies do not work, you could consider a completely or partially electrically operated bed or mattress, but really you should seek advice from your occupational therapist, and/or Social Services Department before embarking on this expensive choice.

As far as turning in bed at night is concerned, this can be quite a problem. There are a number of minor adjustments you can make that may help, after checking the softness of the mattress. Changing your bedclothes or nightdress or pyjamas might help. Some people find that silky bedclothes allow them to turn much more easily than other fabrics. Night socks might also help you get a grip to turn over. A more expensive solution is to purchase a special mattress that assists turning, if these other strategies do not work.

There may be additional problems here that require a different solution: how often do you need to get out of bed during the night to go to the toilet? If this is excessive or difficult, then consult your GP or neurologist to see if some solution, in the form of medication or otherwise, can be found for this.

Kitchen aids

Many people in the household gather in the kitchen and a very diverse range of activities go on there, so it is often worrying when mobility or dexterity problems arise. It is still likely that women will be the main users of the kitchen, despite apparent changes in social attitudes and the household division of labour. However, increasingly other household members like to undertake some tasks in the kitchen, and so it is important to ensure that several household members can use the kitchen easily. It is possible to adapt a kitchen completely for a person with MS, but in a sense this can create problems for other users. In effect, by enabling one person, you can disable others.

Design

If you are starting from scratch, or have decided on a major change in your kitchen area, then the main considerations are likely to be:

- accessibility
- safety
- ease of use, and
- whether other users of the area will be affected.

Obviously the height of worktops and the sink area, especially if you are in a wheelchair, are important considerations. Think about arrangement and access to cupboards, storage areas and cooking facilities, so that you have to move as little as possible, especially if you are likely to be carrying things from one place to another. If you are not yet using a wheelchair, it would still be sensible to think of possible problems when you are making major changes – consider overhanging worktops, for example, so that they can be used from a seated position. Some kitchen systems allow for adjustment with changing circumstances: seek advice from your occupational therapist or specialist kitchen manufacturer about what is available.

The point at which you decide to, or indeed have to, make some major changes in your kitchen area varies so much between individuals and the household situation, that it is difficult to make hard and fast rules about when you should embark on them. Other factors will be critical, particularly resources, and whether you can get additional financial help for such alterations from your local Social Services Department, usually through your occupational therapist.

Food preparation and cooking

There are two broad ways to look at this issue. The first way focuses on using foods which are pre-prepared in various forms, thus minimizing the amount of food preparation that you or members of your household have to undertake. There has been a revolution in this area over the last few years, leading to a major increase in prepared foods, instigated by changing lifestyles and the vastly increased number of women who are undertaking several jobs at once, both inside and outside the home.

Although almost all people, and especially women, feel that they may be neglecting their families by using the staggeringly wide range of convenience foods, many now use such food increasingly to save time and energy. If people with MS do the same, they are not doing anything unusual, but just following a general trend. Many of those foods that are harder for people with mobility problems to prepare – potatoes, salads and vegetables, for example – can now all be purchased in pre-prepared form. Although there is an additional price to pay for these foods, and maybe a minor loss in nutrition, this is more than compensated for by the saving in time and energy that is spent preparing everything yourself – just like most people without MS! You have to strike a balance between convenience and possible modest drawbacks in terms of nutrition. If you are worried about any nutritional issues, you should consult your doctor, or ask for a referral to a dietitian or nutritionist.

The second way is to consider additional aids and equipment that may be available to help you in the kitchen area. These may range from things like non-slip mats to secure mixing bowls, to high stools to work on, special trolleys, and padded handles to ensure a better grip. A wide range of everyday kitchenware, such as knives, forks, spoons, ladles, and so on, are now available in a form that will help you get a better grip. You will quickly find those aids that help you most. Try and phase what you do, so that you do not feel exhausted from working overlong on single tasks without a break. Look for special recipe books that not only suggest nutritious foods, but also show short cuts in food preparation.

Using a microwave oven, especially the modern combination types, can be easier than a conventional one and, although it can be seen as just another short cut, cooking interesting food in such an oven can be quite a challenge. One of the additional benefits of a microwave oven is that it generates less external heat than a conventional oven and this could be an important point for people with MS who are very sensitive to heat.

There is another issue here in relation to cooking and that is safety. Many people with MS have a problem with grip or sensation, and this, together with a hot food or utensil, is not a recommended combination! It is important to keep your eyes on whatever you are carrying, and to use this as a double check to ensure that you are carrying it firmly enough. By and large you should hold things with both hands, rather than with one or two fingers. Choose cups, for example, with two handles, or at least one large handle. In particular, try to carry hot liquids in containers with fitted lids so that, if you do drop them, there is less danger. Wearing rubber or special kitchen gloves can be helpful. For the most part, carrying and holding things is just a question of getting used to the changes in your sensations and grip, and being deliberate and careful about moving things, especially items that are hot.

Writing aids

Conventional pens and pencils are amongst the most difficult items to use if you have problems with grip, or indeed tremor. Pens or pencils that are much bigger in diameter than normal ones and have a less smooth surface are becoming fashionable now because they are ergonomically better for everyone's fingers, and you should be able to find a selection of these in a large stationery shop or suppliers of products for people with disabilities. You could try putting elastic bands around pens and pencils to make them easier to use.

The issue of tremor is in some ways more complex: it is of limited use being able to grip a pen if your writing is such that people have difficulty in reading it. This problem can be managed by weighting your wrist, for example, or by using weighted pens etc., which may dampen down the tremor. However, there is still a problem if you do not have much strength in your wrist. In this case there are various devices, writing guides for example, which help you to form letters and words, lessening the effect of the tremor. You will have to experiment to see if you can find ways of reducing the effect of both lack of grip and of tremor to produce sufficiently good results to be read by others.

Computers

A computer can be costly to buy and costly in terms of the time and effort of training yourself to use it to the full. One of the difficulties at present is the very rapid change in computer systems. No sooner has one been bought than the next – 'enhanced', 'better', 'faster' – model takes its place. It is an industry geared to continuous change, and it is quite likely that the computer you have just bought will be 'out of date' almost immediately. So you need to think very carefully about what you might want to use a computer for, how easy it is to use, and what support will you have in terms of help with programmes or the machine itself, if you get stuck. It would be good idea, if you have a friend with a computer, to check out how easy it is for you to use – in terms of the screen, keyboard and 'mouse'. (Most systems operate with this small matchbox-sized object, which you hold, move and 'click' with a finger to give on-screen commands, although there are other keyboards that do not need the mouse.) This will enable you to see whether you can control the computer easily and have the dexterity to do so. You could think of learning to use a computer as a bit of a challenge!

There are an increasing number of ways in which computers can be controlled even if you do not have the dexterity to use a keyboard or a mouse. There are various pointing devices which can be used. There has also been very rapid progress in voice-activated computer systems in recent years, and some of these can adapt to individual voices even when, as a result of the MS, words may not be formed exactly as they should – or are slurred in some way. However, if the way you say words is changing a lot, then this can be a problem because you may have 'to train' the computer yet again to recognize your voice. In this respect you should investigate the resources available at specialist Communication Aids Centres (see Chapter 9), regarding not only communication itself, but also the many innovative ways in which people with a range of disabilities can both use, and control, computer systems.

Increasingly there are local classes being run for older or disabled people in the use of computers, and even if you cannot get to them, you may be able to talk to someone who runs the classes for advice. You might be able to get a trial run; then seek independent advice about what machine and software you should buy – and especially what support you will receive afterwards. Salesmen for particular machines can be very convincing, and you should not just rely on their advice. This is why you should always try and seek advice from someone you know or a specialist centre, who will understand both what you want to use a computer for and be familiar with the problems that you may have. Of course, there are all kinds of more exotic things you can do with a suitable computer, including using the internet – the World Wide Web for information and communication – sending and receiving faxes or emails, and doing a whole range of things other than writing a letter using a word processing package. However, you should be realistic about what you are likely to be able to do. Some people get addicted and it becomes their life, but for others the computer stays in the corner with hardly any use.

If you have children, particularly older children, they are probably already using computers and would like nothing better than to demonstrate their skills at the expense of their parents!

Help around the house

The issue of housework can be difficult one, particularly for women; despite lots of changes in attitudes, 'keeping a good home' is still a commonplace expectation, even if it is not so openly stated now. For a woman whose life has been in the home, or who is now largely confined to home having given up a job, keeping the house clean and tidy may be something that both she – and perhaps others – see as an indication of her 'usefulness', and, thinking about housework in another way, it is good exercise. It can then be a wrench, even for women who do not care for housework at all, to lose even routine household tasks. For all these reasons, retaining even a very modest range of household activities is important, to feel that you are contributing to the household overall.

A couple of things might help here:

- Arrange things in your house as comfortably and safely as possible for yourself and others in your household. You may then have to compromise over who arranges what room, as long as you have the least disruptive pattern of furniture that you need to be able to move around safely.
- There is a range of equipment that you can use from a standing position, or even at a distance from a sitting position, and this may allow you to do a little at a time, although the heavier jobs, and particularly those which involve moving around equipment – like vacuum cleaners – may need to be undertaken by others, unless you are very careful. You should be able to get further advice from your OT about available equipment and finding ways of managing to do at least some of the housework yourself.

There is more discussion about housing and home adaptations in Chapter 14.

Driving

Benefits available

There are a number of benefits for which you may be eligible. If you receive the higher rate mobility allowance, you will be allowed to claim exemption from vehicle excise duty (road tax) on one vehicle. This exemption is given on condition that the vehicle is used 'solely for the purposes of the disabled person'. Nevertheless, it is likely that some commonsense latitude will be given.

If you have the higher rate mobility allowance, you will be automatically eligible for the Blue Badge, which gives parking privileges, and also for access to the Motability Scheme (see below). You will also get VAT exemption on adaptations to make your car suitable, as well as exemption on the repair, maintenance or replacement of these adaptations.

Motability Scheme

The Department of Transport has set up a Mobility Advice and Vehicle Information Service (MAVIS) to help people choose an appropriate car for their needs, and they will be able to give advice and assistance (see Appendix 1). This advice will cover appropriate vehicles and adaptations, as well as issues concerned with your suitability to drive – an issue that may concern many people with MS, especially in so far as eyesight may be affected, as well as the arm and leg movements necessary to control the vehicle, for which additional technical assistance may be needed.

For people with MS who are receiving the higher rate mobility component of the Disability Living Allowance (DLA), the Motability Scheme can offer a good approach to the purchase of a new car, good used car or an electric wheelchair, through hire purchase. Alternatively, you can hire a car through the same scheme.

Getting into and out of a car – possible adaptations

One of the major problems for a disabled person is swinging round from outside the car into a passenger, or a driver's seat, and of course getting out of the car in the same way. Depending on how much you want to spend, and exactly what your needs are, you could think either of a swivel cushion placed on the seat so that you can swing your legs into the car; or, more elaborately (and more expensively), replacing whole seats and their fittings so that the seat itself swivels; this allows you to back on to the seat from outside, or to rise from the seat to a standing position without having to manoeuvre in and out of the car.

Ability to drive

Licence

You do have to notify the DVLA (Driver Vehicle and Licensing Agency) that you have MS, as it is one of the conditions that may affect your driving ability. If you contact them, you will receive a form PK1 (Application for Driving Licence/Notification of Driving Licence Holder's State of Health) to complete and return. These forms may be available at your local Post Office. When it assesses your application, the DVLA will normally adopt a positive view, for it wishes to give drivers with a current or potential disability the best chance possible of keeping their licences – the key issue in this respect is public safety.

Especially if you have been recently diagnosed, you are unlikely to lose your licence. The DVLA will consider the information that you have given on the form (PK1) and, if it believes that your driving ability is not a hazard to other road users, it will normally issue a 3-year licence. Your situation will be reviewed at the end of these 3 years. If you answer positively to any of the questions concerning health problems on form PK1, then you should send a covering letter explaining your situation, and why you believe that you are fit to drive. Without such a letter or explanation, the DVLA might withdraw your licence. It would also be worth talking to your doctor – GP or neurologist – about your driving ability. If they disagree with you about your capacity to drive, or between themselves, or you yourself have concerns about your driving ability, then you should arrange for an assessment at one of the special driving and mobility assessment centres, which you can find via the Department of Transport's Mobility Advice and Vehicle Information Service (MAVIS) (see Appendix 1).

Judging your ability to drive

Doctors consider driving ability in relation to problems with the use of your arms and legs, your eyesight or your reactions. It is clearly a matter of judgement by the GP or neurologist as to whether any of these or other consequences of MS do indeed affect your driving ability and, of course, one of the main problems with MS is its variability. One day you might be able to drive without any difficulty at all. On another day, through the onset of specific symptoms, it might be difficult, or unsafe, for you to do so. The problem both for you and your doctor is making a reasonable judgement.

Driving a car may well be a lifeline for you. The key issue will be safety for you and other road users. Some other adaptations mentioned earlier might help you to continue driving. So, discuss the issue with your family and friends, and with people in the MS Society (see Appendix 1), who will be able to offer both support and information. In the end, the formal and probably best way to deal with the problem has to be through a driving assessment through a mobility assessment centre. During this assessment, not only your driving ability but also any vehicle adaptations will be considered. The driving assessment centre will write a report – this could be of particular value if, for example, the DVLA decides to rescind your licence, and you decide to appeal against the decision. There is a charge for a driving assessment and this may vary depending on the type of assessment required, so it is important to find out the cost when you arrange it.

Appealing against a licence withdrawal

There is an appeals procedure, but it can be lengthy and complex, and you need to seek advice and consider the likelihood of success, as well as the consequences of not succeeding. In any case, if you feel that you want to appeal, it is important that you register your intent to appeal to the DVLA as soon as possible. In the case of England and Wales, this has to be done within 6 months from the date of notification of the withdrawal of the licence, and in Scotland within 1 month of that date. You can withdraw your intent to appeal at any time. Appeals are heard in the local Magistrates Court in England and Wales, and in the Sheriff's Court in Scotland.

You will almost certainly need some formal assistance to appeal, and you ought to bear in mind that it will be difficult to succeed without supporting evidence from your doctor and/or your formal driving assessment, which may not have been available to the DVLA at the time the original decision was made. It would be sensible to consult with someone who has experience of such cases, perhaps the Citizens Advice, your local DIAL (Disability Information and Advice Line) or your local branch of the MS Society who could refer you on to others, even a good lawyer, if necessary. Look in your local telephone book for their addresses. It is salutary to know that the DVLA has often in the past sought to recover its expenses from those who have appealed unsuccessfully, and this could amount to several hundred pounds. So you need to very sure of your grounds before appealing.

Telling the insurance company

Your insurance company cannot stop you holding a driving licence – only the DVLA or the Courts can do that. However, insurance companies do require that you disclose all material factors that may affect your driving. MS is one of these factors. If you do not disclose the information, this may invalidate your insurance and, if you are not insured (at least on a third-party basis), you are not allowed to drive. So it is essential to tell your insurance company about your MS because, if you do not and then a legitimate claim arises which has nothing to do with the MS, you may find that you are in difficulty.

Generally, as long as you have a valid driving licence, the most significant problem that you may face is a slightly increased insurance premium. Ask for several quotations from a number of companies to make sure that you are getting the best value. You also ought to read the small print on any policy proposal because you may need to be wary of unacceptable or difficult endorsements to the policy.

You could also contact some of the insurance companies who are now specializing in insuring disabled drivers. A list is obtainable through RADAR (*Mobility Fact Sheet No.6*), which sets out these companies, and broadly what they offer (see Appendix 2). You might even lower your premium!

Other transport

We have already discussed the possibility of getting an outdoor electric wheelchair or an electric scooter (sometimes called pavement vehicles) which, depending on the terrain near where you live, could be of great help in giving you more independence and ability to travel reasonable distances for shopping or leisure activities.

There are other forms of transport that you may find helpful, but these tend to vary according to which area you are living in. You can get in touch with the Social Services Department of your local authority for advice.

- There are **Dial-a-Ride minibus schemes**, especially for people with mobility problems. Often you have to join the scheme first, and there might be a waiting list. However, when you have joined, you will be collected from your home and then dropped back again, often at a reasonable cost.
- Some areas have **taxi voucher schemes** that give a number of low or no-cost journeys. These are usually in operation where people cannot take advantage of free or concessionary bus fares. Although taxi fares generally can be expensive, sometimes people do not realize how expensive maintaining a car is, and you could find that using taxis for short journeys compares very favourably.
- For longer journeys outside your area, there are organizations such as **Tripscope**, which can help you plan such journeys, and from whom you may be able to obtain escorts if necessary.
- Sometimes, **other organizations**, such as St John Ambulance Brigade and the British Red Cross, and local organizations and clubs, such as Rotary, Lions, Round Table and the Soroptomists can also provide escorts. Have a look in your local telephone book for their addresses.
- Your **local MS Society branch** or region may be able to help.

9
Speech difficulties

Such things as facial expression, body movement and gesture are all linked with speech, in order to communicate our thoughts and needs. Nevertheless, it is speech itself which is often the focus of concern. As with other symptoms of MS, problems with speech can vary, particularly in the earlier stages of the disease. Although the problem cannot currently be remedied by curing the neurological problem, appropriate advice, support and exercises can improve things considerably.

Voice production

Voice production is a complicated process involving coordination between the relevant muscle groups, which in normal life (without MS or other condition affecting voice production) we tend to take for granted. Speech problems are normally assessed by speech therapists – they need to know just where the problem lies for management:

- **Breathing**: You may not be able to exhale in a slow and measured enough way needed for good speech production.
- **Phonation**: You may not be able to speak loudly enough or with sufficient clarity or tone of voice.
- **Resonance**: This additional quality of sound may be hampered by your palate not working properly.
- **Articulation**: Your vocal movements may not be sufficiently precise to articulate sounds properly.
- **Phrasing and continuity**: You may have difficulty in putting all the sounds together to produce sentences with appropriate pauses and so on.

Sometimes speech may be 'scanning', which means that each syllable is pronounced as if it is a separate word. Occasionally speech may be 'explosive/staccato', where a syllable is forced out in a loud manner. Both these problems arise when MS affects the 'cerebellum', the part of the brain that deals with coordination.

Each of these areas can be affected by particular combinations of defective muscle control.

If you can manage your level of fatigue well, and reduce or shorten the effects of exacerbations or attacks of MS, you may find that you have fewer problems with your speech. However, this will not always be the case and, of course, if the MS progresses, it is more likely that problems with speech will arise at some point.

As far as the sound and tone of your voice is concerned, these change in any case as we grow older, which is why it is generally quite easy to recognize the voice of a child as different from that of an older person. In MS different aspects of voice production may change more quickly as the disease affects the various muscles of the face, mouth and throat in different ways. Because of the damage to muscle control, your voice may be more difficult to control – it may sound high or low quite suddenly, or your speech may not sound very smooth, or perhaps you may lose your voice in mid-sentence. These problems are mainly caused by the varying, and sometimes sudden, changes in the way that your nervous system is transmitting messages to this sophisticated and normally coordinated system of voice production. There is little that can be done for the neurological difficulty itself. It is mainly a question of being aware of the problems that you have, as well as pacing your speech, and exercising the muscles to try and retain their maximum use for as long as possible.

Dysarthria

When people speak it requires considerable coordination of a large number of facial and related muscles. Your speech may slur because the normal muscular control of voice production has failed through weakness, or because the muscles are not operating in the right sequence. As a result your speech may sound slurred or be uncoordinated. 'Dysarthria' is the name given to general problems like this and may be associated with several neurological diseases. Sometimes your speech will just sound slightly slurred, but still be intelligible to others, but with more serious problems of coordination it may be difficult for others to understand you.

Helping yourself

The first thing is to be aware of when your speech is unclear or slurred. Ask others sympathetically to understand what your problem is. People tend to do things more quickly nowadays, and seem to have less patience with others, who may not keep up with their fast pace. This is true even in family settings. Tell people that you are not drunk or have anything wrong with your mental state, just a problem of coordination of your voice.

Check how long people have the time to talk with you, so that you are not disappointed if they leave in the middle of a conversation. When people understand your situation, they will be willing to spend more time in conversation with you. You can help also by:

- being much more deliberate in your speech;
- trying to pronounce your words much more precisely;
- slowing down your normal pace of speech, and
- giving yourself more time by pausing periodically.

Through these means you can maintain a good rhythm, even if you speak much more slowly than you would normally.

Learn to breathe in ways that assist the production of speech – coordinated breathing in sequence with your speech is crucial.

Don't try and speak for too long as this could exacerbate the problems with your speech, and both you and your friends may 'lose the thread' of what you are saying. After all some of the most memorable or amusing things that we hear are very short and to the point!

Further help

Communication technology is advancing rapidly. The newer computer voice recognition programmes are still very expensive but are improving quickly. Some other computerized systems may be of help but, before you think of high technology solutions, many much simpler devices and procedures may be better, including such things as:

- picture or word charts;
- alphabet charts where you can spell out the words that you want with your fingers or eyes;
- agreed signals with your partner/family/friends for yes, no and other words, or
- eye blink systems.

Your choice is likely to be influenced by your own skills, how comfortable you and others feel with a particular system, and the costs (financial and otherwise) that your choice may incur.

If you are buying a computer, get independent advice on which system is the most appropriate for you. Think about the future also before you buy because computer systems quickly become outdated! There are currently systems, portable as well as desk-top, that automatically print out your messages and translate your words into speech. Some allow you to use single key strokes, not only to create more complex messages but to control other facilities around the home. It is not possible to give individual advice to you here, because of the rapid changes occurring, as well as because everyone's abilities and needs are so personal. A range of communication aids can be supplied by the statutory services depending on your circumstances, including your local education authority, NHS Trusts, GP fund holders, and the Department of Employment; there are also Communication Aids Centres, in addition to individual professional advice. You should ask your GP, neurologist or occupational or speech therapist for a referral to a specialist centre if possible.

10
Eating and swallowing difficulties; diet and nutrition

Issues centred on food and nutrition, including both what you eat and how it is eaten, can become a major preoccupation of people with MS, especially if the disease progresses. Some of the concerns relate to the most appropriate diet for someone with MS, and others relate to the swallowing mechanism, which can be affected in a range of ways in MS. Although many people do not develop swallowing difficulties – it depends very much on the particular areas in which demyelination has taken place – when there are problems, they can be difficult to manage easily.

Eating and swallowing difficulties

Some people have major difficulty in swallowing! There are a number of different causes for this difficulty (the medical term is 'dysphagia'), depending on exactly which muscles are affected in the journey of food and drink from the mouth to the stomach. Problems might be linked to the chewing process, or to the muscles that push the food or drink towards the throat, or to those muscles that coordinate the swallowing process through the throat and oesophagus to the stomach. Of course, there may be other problems, such as food particles remaining in the mouth that could create problems in breathing, for food particles can accidentally get into the airways to the lung. However, normally, the problems that people with MS experience are ones related to delays in the swallowing process, and a slowing down of the passage of food and drink through the throat area.

You may also have difficulty in swallowing liquids, especially those that are less viscous and 'dense'. This is because the liquids pass through the mouth 'too fast' before the slower moving muscles have a chance to coordinate swallowing, so you may end up coughing and choking, as liquids run into your airway to your lungs. Usually this problem is solved by thickening the liquids, so that they pass through your mouth more slowly.

Professional help with swallowing

As soon as you notice any difficulties with swallowing, it is worth asking the advice of your GP or neurologist at this early stage. They will refer you to a therapist for further advice and support. Increasingly there are more formal evaluations of swallowing problems in order to try and understand exactly where the problems lie. Sometimes this assessment may include what is called 'videofluoroscopy', which allows the process of your swallowing to be seen on X-ray following a barium swallow. Occasionally it may also include an endoscopic examination – this involves passing a small fibreoptic tube through and past the throat so that additional information can be obtained. Professional help for swallowing difficulties centres on teaching exercises to try and:

- strengthen your muscles involved in swallowing;
- enhance the coordination of your breathing and swallowing (so as to avoid choking);
- strengthen the muscles controlling your lips and tongue that help in managing the food in your mouth in preparation for swallowing.

Self-help in relation to swallowing

It is possible to give general guidelines as to what you can do yourself to help swallowing, although it must be remembered each person has slightly different problems, and thus not every strategy will work for everyone. However, things to try yourself include:

- changing the type and preparation of your food – solid foods, particularly those that are only half chewed, are much more difficult to swallow than those which are softer, so you may need to consider chopping or blending food;
- changing the ways in which you eat and swallow – eating little and often may help;
- exercising to strengthen the relevant muscles as much as possible;
- making sure that you do not talk (or laugh) and eat at the same

time – problems of swallowing can often be linked to trying to do two things at once!

* being careful in drinking liquids – in fact, trying to make a runny liquid thicker (more 'viscous'), similar to the consistency of a thick milkshake.

Managing saliva

For most people, dealing with saliva is virtually automatic. You salivate and swallow the saliva almost without thinking. In MS, coordination of the swallowing reflex with the amount of saliva you have may become a problem. You may begin to notice what appear to be large amounts of saliva. It is not that you are producing more saliva, but the swallowing of it becomes far more noticeable. In general you have to become more conscious of the process of swallowing, and try and systematically swallow. Indeed swallowing exercises may help you and, paradoxically, by stimulating more regular production of salivation through sucking a sweet (preferably sugar free!) can also help in ensuring that you swallow regularly.

A problem often arises when you 'forget' to swallow for a period of time and then suddenly notice the saliva. You might try a sequence of events as you eat or drink a little at a time, based on the following: 'Hold your breath, swallow, clear your throat, then swallow again.'

Choking

Those who do have serious problems swallowing with MS are always worried about choking. Mostly this can be managed by following the suggestions earlier. Some people still have great difficulty but, if food or drink gets into your lungs, which could possibly lead to pneumonia, then more drastic action may be required. The time being taken to eat and drink may also be now so substantial that you run the risk of not getting adequate nutrition or liquids over a period of time. If this happens, then you may find yourself losing weight, getting weaker and having further problems. It is an important decision to move from normal feeding by mouth (oral feeding and drinking) to non-oral feeding, where food is directly channelled into the stomach (often avoiding the mouth and swallowing completely), but this step may be necessary if problems with nutrition and/or concern over choking becomes substantial.

Non-oral feeding

The best way to consider changing to non-oral feeding is to think about it as being a temporary move. For example, after certain kinds of surgery in hospital, not associated with MS, people may be fed on a short-term basis through a tube that passes through the nose and then through the throat directly to the stomach (a 'nasogastric tube'). This particular kind of arrangement has to be temporary because the throat and nose may become irritated after a while. A more long-term arrangement is to have a PEG ('percutaneous endoscopic gastrostomy') in which a tube is inserted through the abdominal wall directly into the stomach. A special feeding formula is regularly pumped through the tube to your stomach. As with any surgical openings through the skin, hygiene is particularly important, and great care has to be taken to prevent infections arising.

Although it is a particularly difficult step to move to non-oral feeding, for social reasons as well as because of the loss of the pleasures associated with normal eating and drinking, in some cases it may be the best decision, in order to build up your strength if you have been losing a lot of weight, and to prevent fears associated with choking. If you are very careful, it may also be possible to continue to eat or drink a few things orally, at least to retain some of the pleasures of eating normally.

You should keep an eye on how your swallowing goes, and always consult with your professional advisors about the possibility of gradually changing the balance between oral and non-oral feeding, so that you can try and resume a greater proportion of oral feeding, with a view to removing the PEG method of feeding if you can. This problem, as with many others in MS, needs constant review.

Diet and nutrition

There are two broad ways in which diet and nutrition can be considered in relation to MS. The first and less contentious relates to your general health: ideas about what is a good diet for general health do, of course, change from time to time. The second deals with the possible beneficial or harmful effects that some diets themselves might have on either symptoms or, more fundamentally, on the underlying cause of the MS.

Diet is the most obvious and easy to implement factor that could be changed by people with MS, and many people have focused on this issue. Also, health care professionals are often very interested in diet and its effects on all aspects of general health. Although there has been research on diet and MS, it has not been a core interest of most researchers because Western populations are largely well-nourished – obesity and overeating, on the contrary, are major health concerns.

There have been many diets that have been suggested to affect either specific symptoms or the cause of MS. There is little evidence that any of these diets has the effects that their supporters suggest – however, we here discuss a number of the more plausible diets.

Essential fatty acids

One of the areas of nutrition that has been researched in relation to MS has been that of 'essential fatty acids', which form part of the building blocks of the brain and nervous system tissue, and are essential to the development and maintenance of the CNS. Actually essential fatty acid is rather an odd phrase in lay terms, for we are used to thinking of anything 'fatty' as very bad for you. However, there are many kinds of 'fats', ranging from the saturated fats, often found in meat and dairy produce, too much of which is not good for you, to the unsaturated and polyunsaturated fats, many of which are found in vegetable sources, and from some of which key essential fatty acids are derived – these are broadly very good for you. About 60% of normal nervous system tissue is made up of these 'essential fatty acids'.

Some research has suggested that several of these essential fatty acids are present in lower quantities in the CNS of people with MS than in that of people without the disease; one theory has been that MS arose because, in their early years such people were deprived of (or unable to assimilate) these essential fatty acids in the development or maintenance of the structure and function of the CNS. However, the reasons for this lower level of fatty acids remain a matter of speculation. Is it a cause or effect of the disease? Does it occur very early in life? Some scientists have thought that the obvious remedy would be to increase the intake of these fatty acids. However, things did not prove to be as simple as that, for many of the essential fatty acids are produced indirectly by the breakdown in the body of particular constituents from the food that we eat.

The use of oil from the evening primrose plant, and some other oils, has become quite common amongst people with MS, for they do provide some of these constituents in a relatively 'purer' form (see Chapter 3 on *Complementary therapies and MS*) but its effectiveness has not been proven scientifically. It is not clear, however, even if the level of the essential fatty acids is returned to 'normal', whether this will affect the course of MS, if the CNS damage has already been under way for some time. Research on this point has not proved conclusive, although many people with MS still feel that, on a precautionary basis, they wish to continue taking these essential oils.

It would not be wise to assume that, if you eat more of the food containing essential fatty acids, it will have a definite and positive effect on your MS or its symptoms. There are several reasons for this:

- The deficiency in essential fatty acids in the brain may be a result of some other process that causes MS; remedying this deficiency may not of itself produce major benefits in relation to the disease.
- The particular fatty acids, often in relatively short supply in the brain tissue of people with MS, are not ones that you can just eat in increased quantity; they are actually produced by the body itself through a conversion process from other less complex fatty acids, and these you can eat. It is this conversion process in the body, which changes simpler forms of fatty acids into more complex ones needed by the brain, that appears to be defective in people with MS. So, even if you have eaten good quantities of the simpler fatty acids, they may not be converted into the vital and more complex ones.
- The process of eating and digestion itself may reduce the amount of the simpler fatty acids being absorbed into the body.
- The relationship between increasing the intake of brain-building fatty acids and the subsequent symptoms of MS is not clear. In principle, whilst more of the fatty acids should assist nervous system function, the relationship between one and the other, and particularly in reducing any symptoms that you might have, appears to be very complex.
- It is likely that any damage to the nervous system from lower levels of essential fatty acids is longstanding, and has occurred, at least in part, very early in life, so it would be very optimistic to expect major changes as a result of a change of diet perhaps several decades later.

Nevertheless, there are a number of studies, not many of them scientifically well designed, which suggest that there may be specific benefits to MS from increasing your intake of those foods that help form complex essential fatty acids, and from decreasing your intake of saturated fats. Although many people believe that this broad strategy can help fight the disease, most scientists and doctors do not.

Which foods are involved?

To get technical for a moment, there are two important families of essential fatty acids for brain function. The first of these is called the 'omega-6 group', with linoleic acid as its 'parent' – the parent meaning the basic fatty acid from which all the others in the family are derived. The second is the 'omega-3 group', with alpha-linoleic acid as its 'parent'. In each case more complex fatty acids are formed in the body from simpler ones. Foods rich in the omega-6 family are those such as:

- sunflower and safflower seed oil
- evening primrose oil
- offal such as liver; kidney, brains, sweetbread
- lean meat
- legumes (peas and beans).

Food rich in the omega-3 family are:

- green vegetables
- fish and seafood
- fish liver oils
- linseeds
- certain legumes.

The difficulty is that most of these foods contain only small quantities of the relevant fatty acids, and then only in their simplest form. However, one or two foods have been found to have not only larger quantities of essential fatty acids, but to have them in a form that is closer to that needed by the brain. For example, the oil of the evening primrose plant has become a very popular dietary supplement for people with MS, because it is unique and contains large quantities of a substance called gamma-linoleic acid, a more complex form of linoleic acid, which is converted into further important fatty acids by the body. Some other rarer oils may also contain good quantities of gamma-linoleic acid.

In principle, the effects of taking these fatty acids could be profound on some key characteristics of the underlying pathology of MS, but in formal clinical trials the results have not been as good as hoped for, although there is some evidence from one or two good trials that attacks of MS may be fewer over time in those taking additional fatty acids. However, these results do not approach the more dramatic findings from studies on the latest immune-based drugs.

Many people with MS continue to take evening primrose oil even if, for example, they do not follow religiously all the other dietary recommendations, either as a kind of 'insurance policy', in that they are doing something that they hope will help the MS, or – and there are reasonable grounds for this – knowing that is not actually harmful, and may be helpful to your general health. It is likely to be a more costly alternative than modifying your diet to include some of the other foods containing essential fatty acids, but may be easier to manage. We must state again that the effectiveness of evening primrose oil has not been proven scientifically.

Saturated fats

People argue about whether changes in your saturated fat intake will make any difference to your MS. If, in general, essential fatty acids are 'good', then you could increase your intake of these as we have noted, and/or reduce your intake of the 'bad' saturated fats. Of course, there are general health grounds for suggesting that you should lower your intake of saturated fats, but some people who have devised low saturated fat diets for their MS claim that such diets may be far more beneficial for their MS. Again, there is little formal evidence that reducing your intake of saturated fats will specifically stabilize or improve your MS.

Exclusion diets

Cutting out saturated fats is an exclusion diet, but there are other diets that cut out many more specific substances. MS symptoms are considered by some people to be an allergic reaction to certain foods or drinks, and this view has led to other exclusion diets. One such diet is the 'gluten-free diet', in which it is argued that gluten has produced damage in the digestive and elimination system and has made the MS worse. Thus by eliminating gluten it is hoped that damage to the intestine can be prevented. Such diets were developed from those for people with coeliac disease who cannot absorb fats when gluten is present from cereal grains. At one stage these diets gained considerable popularity, but the burden placed on people with MS to stick to a very rigid gluten-free diet, together with disappointing results for many people and a lack of scientific support, has led to their decline.

The relative success claimed for very different diets in particular individuals suggests not so much that these diets are improving MS, but that concomitant problems are possibly being helped in some way by the diets. Of course, if your general health is better, you will feel better, and certain (but not all) symptoms of your MS might be a little improved. The key issue is balancing whatever benefits that you may be gaining against the costs, time and resources that you have to devote to maintaining what can be a formidable dietary regimen.

A healthy diet

There are certain general dietary principles now widely accepted for general health which, on those grounds alone, should be considered by people with MS. These include:

- very little intake of saturated fat (with very limited dairy produce, and generally only certain specific cuts of meat, liver for example);
- plenty of fish;
- a plentiful intake of vegetables and salads – either raw or as lightly cooked as possible;
- pulses;
- plenty of fresh fruit;
- a good intake of most nuts, seeds and seed oils (but excluding those containing saturated oils and certain nuts containing saturated fats, such as brazil nuts);
- as little as possible refined carbohydrates, sugar, processed or packaged foods;
- cutting down on alcohol consumption, and
- cutting out smoking.

In addition, if you want to supplement this diet with liver and/or evening primrose oil, for example, it will not do you any harm, as long as you don't feel these supplements are adding greatly to your budget.

Most of these recommendations are broadly in line with more general nutritional advice for a healthy lifestyle, although they may be rather more draconian in relation to eating meat, for example than those general diets. So, even if you do not believe the various claims – some verging on the miraculous – that have been made by individuals for the diets devised for themselves or for their partners with MS, there are good grounds for following the broad guidelines. You may feel healthier on this kind of diet just because your general health might have improved. If symptoms of your MS have been helped, that would be a bonus.

Vitamin and mineral supplements

Most of the diets used by people with MS appear to be also supplemented by various vitamins and minerals. The value of these for MS itself is unclear, although there is a mountain of popular information suggesting that most vitamins and minerals in our bodies need supplementing. However, there is little scientific evidence that the average healthy adult with a reasonably balanced diet needs any significant vitamin or mineral supplements. The key questions for people with MS are:

- How much has your general health been compromised and do you need supplementation for this?
- Will additional vitamins and minerals help your MS?

As far as general health is concerned, it is clearly important that people with MS receive a balanced intake of vitamins and minerals appropriate to their age, gender and situation. This can best be undertaken through a balanced diet, of the general kind we have mentioned above. Supplementation should only be necessary where, for various reasons, it is not possible to follow such a diet. There is little scientific evidence that supplementing beyond this general level will produce significant health benefits, although many popular books appear to suggest so.

Vitamin supplements

There is no scientific evidence that serious deficiencies in vitamin intake could produce the kind of damage in the nervous system evident in MS. So, conversely, the key question is whether major supplementation could produce beneficial effects. Since the 1920s there have been claims that supplementation with various vitamins (A, B_1, B_6, B_{12}, C, D, E, K) singly and in combination, administered by mouth, injection or intraspinally, have had some beneficial effect on MS. Most of these studies have not been controlled against a group of people with MS who did not take the vitamins and, for various other reasons, the studies have been scientifically dubious.

Although some of the studies suggest the benefits of vitamin supplementation, it is likely that most of these benefits were the result of the often spontaneous and unpredictable changes in the course of MS, and not the vitamins themselves. High dose 'megavitamin' therapy has also become relatively popular. Although there are many anecdotal reports of changes in MS, there is still no reliable scientific evidence that 'megadoses' of any vitamin or vitamin combinations have any effect on the course of the disease. The administration of vitamins A and D, in particular, has to be undertaken carefully as they are toxic in high doses. Vitamin B_6 may also produce symptoms in the peripheral nervous system at high doses, and vitamin C can produce stomach problems and kidney stones.

Overall, the formal evidence on vitamins and MS suggests that, apart from taking care that you have a normal balanced intake of vitamins, there is little to be gained from major supplementation of vitamins in your diet.

Mineral supplements

A broadly similar position seems to apply here. Many minerals have been tried in MS over the years. These have ranged from gold, silver, mercury, arsenic, thorium, metallic salts and potassium bromide to, more recently, manganese, zinc and potassium gluconate. There is a paradox that some of the metals tested earlier, for example mercury, can produce neurological symptoms themselves. The more recent candidates are generally based on a sounder principles, but they have not, for the most part, been subjected to careful evaluation through formal scientific studies.

There is a problem in devising effective vitamin or mineral therapies, even if it is accepted that there is a key role for minerals and vitamins in MS, in that how the body uses them is poorly understood. Often it is not the presence of a major dose of some mineral or vitamin that is the key, but the fact that they all work in a complex way together. Also, many mineral and vitamin supplements are not taken in a form that the body can easily use, and are in any case changed, as in the case of essential fatty acids, into the different substances needed by the body. This is why it is far better, if possible, to eat a balanced diet rather than go to the expense of supplements.

In general, there is little evidence that major doses of any minerals or vitamins will help MS, and a number – indeed perhaps most – are toxic when used in large doses, and produce neurological symptoms themselves.

Nutrition and weight reduction

This can be a problem for all or us! As we grow older, everyone tends to put on more body weight, unless we become increasingly careful about what we eat and how we exercise. When you are in a wheelchair, or are sitting down most of the day, clearly you are likely to get less exercise than you used to do. Lack of exercise together with a fondness for processed carbohydrates and getting a little older, produces the weight gain. It can be tackled in a number of ways, but for anyone who has evolved a lifestyle – whether by force or design – that has led to weight increase, it is not an easy task to take it off again.

In seeking to reduce weight it is important to tackle the problem sensibly. Just eating very little is not necessarily the right solution, for your diet must be a balanced one. It is also important to bear in mind that almost all weight loss achieved very quickly is put back on again within a short period of time.

Even more concerning, in the case of multiple sclerosis, is that in rapid weight loss, a proportion, and sometimes a substantial proportion can involve loss of muscle tissue, even when people are considerably overweight – this is the last thing that people with MS should be risking.

Thus it is important to have a long-term plan of weight loss in which you should not aim to lose much more than a pound a week. This steady loss of weight is less likely to be put on again quickly, and it will not risk muscle loss in the same way as very rapid weight loss. You ought to try and get back to a diet with less processed carbohydrates and more fresh fruit and vegetables. By and large vegetables are bulky but have far less carbohydrates, including saturated fats, than processed foods. It may mean a bit of painful adaptation as you change from sweet, sugary and fat-based foods to others, but it is worth the effort. Perhaps one of the most important things is to try and make this a family affair for you and your partner, friend or children. Food eating is a social activity and being a successful dieter often involves not just getting the moral support of others, but their joining in with you. It will be good for them as well!

As far as exercise is concerned, there are more things than you usually think that you can do if you are in a wheelchair. You should ask your physiotherapist in particular what exercises you can do. Find out about any classes you could join at local sports and leisure centres: they are increasing in popularity, again on the principle that group support is important in maintaining exercise. Chapter 8 discusses exercising in more detail.

In general, losing weight is easier if you have other things to do, and are not thinking about food as the main highlight of your day. Good luck!

11
Eyesight and hearing problems

Problems with vision are very common with MS. More than 80% of people with MS experience visual problems at some point. These problems can arise from damage caused by MS to many different pathways of the visual system. Eye movement abnormalities can also develop as a result of this damage. Thus it is important to acknowledge that eye problems are very likely to be the result of MS and to seek support on this basis. However, eyesight problems can occur for many other reasons than MS – people may have short or long sight or other visual problems, for which glasses or contact lenses will be useful and, as people age, some of these problems will become more evident. So be sure to have these problems, and those specifically caused by the MS itself, checked out.

Eyesight

Optic neuritis

What is called optic neuritis is probably the most common visual symptom of MS, perhaps appears in 50% of people with MS, and indeed may well appear before any other symptoms of the disease are obvious. Optic neuritis (inflammation of the optic nerve, which is at the back of the eye) may result in various kinds of vision loss or difficulty. The acute form may result in temporary loss or disturbance of vision in one eye, and very occasionally vision loss at the same time in both eyes – although one eye may follow the other in being affected. Vision loss or disturbance may most often be in the centre of the eye, but it may also be in peripheral vision. Chronic optic neuritis can result in a range of continuing visual symptoms. Even those people with normal sharpness of vision (visual acuity) may have a reduced capacity to deal with contrasts in their visual field, or have reduced colour vision.

When such a symptom appears, it can be a very worrying development for people with MS – as can be expected in anyone if a sudden loss of vision occurs. In almost all cases vision reappears and is often almost back to normal after a period of time. However, this process may take several weeks. Symptoms of optic neuritis can worsen for up to 2 weeks after its initial onset, then most people recover rapidly and have improved back to their pre-attack state after 5 weeks. Recovery in a very few cases may take up to a year. Some people who have had an attack may feel that the quality of their vision is not quite as it was, and they can be left with some problems in relation to colour vision, depth perception and contrast sensitivity. Optic neuritis can also be present without any obvious major symptoms, although on careful checking minor abnormalities can often be detected in such cases.

It is important to say that there are a range of other conditions that may result in condiditons similar to optic neuritis. In relation to MS itself there is strong link between the presence of optic neuritis and the disease in the form of CNS lesions – mostly the larger the number of lesions detected by MRI the more likely MS is the cause.

Treating optic neuritis

Corticosteroids have been the main basis of medical treatment for optic neuritis for some time, even though there is conflicting research about the effectiveness of their use. The basis of the use of these drugs is that they have some effect on the immune system. In relation to what can be described as inflammatory eye disease, it is thought they could help in reducing the inflammation. A combination of methylprednisolone and prednisone may be given, although this may vary. Because in most cases (even the most severe), vision returns to something like its previous state in a reasonable period of time, some neurologists are reluctant to give powerful steroid drugs, which can have significant side effects. So, although it is worrying for people with a sudden onset of these symptoms, waiting for the return of vision or the lessening of visual disturbances is often the strategy that is followed.

With the advent of beta-interferon type drugs in MS (where optic neuritis can be one symptom), there has been increasing pressure to give such drugs at an earlier stage in the condition. In principle, if the MS could be detected earlier – and optic neuritis is a frequent symptom occurring before MS has been diagnosed – then optic neuritis would probably be a symptom that responded to such a treatment. However, definitively diagnosing MS at such an early stage may not be easy, and there is still much debate about how appropriate the beta-interferons are to give to all people at that stage of MS.

Eye movement abnormalities

Eye movement abnormalities are quite common in MS. These can take many forms depending on the nature of the neurological damage. They might involve rapid but regular eye movements (usually described as 'nystagmus') or take a range of other forms including a temporarily fixed gaze. Many of these abnormal movements may not even be recognized by the person with MS, and are more likely to be noticed by others. Occasionally people with MS experience a more troubling form of nystagmus, which involves very slow but regular eye movements associated sometimes with dizziness and nausea. Nystagmus is a difficult condition to treat successfully, for the damage that causes it can be very different in different cases. Clonazepam (Rivotril) can sometimes help the problem, as can baclofen or gabapentin and scopolamine, although it is often a case of trial and error in their use.

Uhtoff's phenomenon

Another occasional symptom is a visual disturbance after exercise, a meal or hot bath ('Uhtoff's phenomenon'), almost certainly due to increased body heat affecting nerve conduction. Such a visual disturbance will normally disappear as body heat falls.

Other sight problems

Although it is unusual for someone with MS to lose their sight completely (even if this is only temporary), many people have episodes during which their sight will become worse. Only one, or both eyes may be affected, and your sight may be disturbed in various ways, including:

- double vision ('diplopia')
- a blank field or spot in the middle of your vision ('scotoma')
- loss of peripheral vision
- blurring of vision
- problems with colour vision, or certain contrasts, such as an unusual balance between light and shade in the visual field
- pain on eye movement from inflammation of the optic nerve.

Visual disturbances may be especially noticeable at night when light is much less, although there may be the impression in daylight of colours being pale or 'washed out'. You may feel you need to leave a light on at night to assist your vision in the evening.

Management

These visual symptoms are not, unfortunately, correctable by glasses or contact lenses, because they are caused by nerve damage or inflammation. Although these disturbances can be very disconcerting, they do usually settle down on their own over hours, days or, occasionally, weeks, but there may be some residual loss of vision over time. Probably the most sensible approach is to wait, if you can, for the visual disturbances to correct themselves. You may be able to deal with the double vision temporarily by putting a patch over one eye, but this strategy will slow the natural adaptation of the brain to double vision. Sometimes prisms placed in glasses can help to reduce the effects of double vision by bringing the two images together. High-dose corticosteroids (such as methylprednisolone or dexamethasone) can clear problems earlier, but like other powerful drugs, they can cause side effects. You will need to be aware that visual problems can increase with fatigue, infection, stress, etc., and so managing these issues will help those visual problems.

Cataracts

Cataracts (clouding of the lens of the eye) may occur more frequently in people with MS partly because they are linked with the extensive use of cortisone treatments, which have been relatively commonly used in MS. Cataracts can, however, be surgically removed and this can result in a substantial improvement in vision.

Hearing problems

MS is not known to cause significant symptoms in hearing (although there can always be the occasional exception), even if a test called an 'auditory evoked response' reveals some damage to the relevant nervous pathways. Very, very occasionally some hearing loss may occur temporarily as a result of the MS but, if your hearing loss is gradual or persistent, it needs investigating for other causes. Sometimes in order to diagnose and help problems with your speech, an audiological assessment may be carried out; however, any problems – as we have noted – are almost certainly not caused by the MS itself.

12
Employment

At the time when men and women are diagnosed with MS, almost all are in employment of some kind. Considering how the diagnosis is going to affect your current job and future career is therefore a matter of considerable importance. Many issues arise in this context, including how or indeed whether to tell your employer; whether it might still be possible to continue work and, if so, on what basis, and what the implications might be financially.

Telling your employer

You need to think this situation through beforehand, and rehearse what you might say. It is very important that your employer knows something about MS before you speak to them if possible. Any negative, or less than positive, reaction to what you say may be due as much to ignorance of MS, as to any particular problem with you personally. The MS Society has produced a helpful leaflet called *Employing People with Multiple Sclerosis – some questions answered*, and this would be worth giving or sending to your employer.

When you are talking to your employer, you must remember that, in terms of his or her response to you, they are thinking in business terms, however much they might like you personally. So it is important that you understand this and present in effect a 'business case' to them. A business case would emphasize your training, experience, commitment and your value to the organization, and would present a realistic – and thus modest – view of the likely problems that you might 'cost' the organization in terms of absence for sickness in the foreseeable future. It would also indicate that your abilities in many areas of your work were unlikely to be affected. If there are minor changes in working practices or additional equipment that you might need, not just to compensate for reduced mobility, for example, but also your productivity and hence your organization's enhancement, then try arguing for them. For many employers, keeping skilled personnel who know the organization and its objectives and clients is more preferable to finding new employees, especially if they are convinced that you will continue to perform well in your job.

Promotion

This is a more difficult issue. Whilst the battle to reduce prejudice against people with MS at work is gradually being won for people in their current jobs, many employers still have a concern about promoting people with the condition. In your current job you will have proved yourself, that is almost certainly why you are applying for promotion, and thus your employer – presumably – is likely to be satisfied with your work in that job. However, he or she may find the combination of your promotion to a new position where you will not yet, of course, have demonstrated your competence, and a condition with variable symptoms, difficult to be positive about. So, if you tell your employer about your MS, you should stress the qualities that you have (unaffected by the MS), and how important these would be for the job you are going after. It may well be that your previous skills and experience are such that a positive decision on promotion is relatively easy.

Telling your colleagues

Given the way that news gets around, it is unlikely that you will be able to tell one colleague without others becoming aware of your situation quite quickly. Despite your wishes, sometimes it can even happen that information from outside your work situation alerts colleagues about your MS unintentionally, for example an inadvertent message from a family member to a colleague about an absence from work. So it is probably wise to work out ways in which to tell your colleagues in a planned process.

Although most of your colleagues will have probably heard something about MS, their views will be based on a wide range of experiences and ideas, and thus may not be accurate. This will not help in the understanding of your condition. So you will need to do more than simply indicating your diagnosis. The best thing may be to give each of your colleagues some written information about MS – perhaps one or more of the pamphlets on MS available from the MS Society – at the time you are informing them about your situation. They can then have accurate information, and you can respond to any questions that they might want to ask you about your own MS. It may be worth reminding them, if they were not aware of your MS before you told them, that this shows how little your work, and your working relationships with them were affected – and indeed this may continue for a long time.

The Disability Discrimination Act 1995 and employment

The provisions of the Disability Discrimination Act 1995 are in principle very substantial, and apply to many aspects of employment. However, the exact implications of many of the provisions have not yet all been legally tested, so it will only become clear over the years how precisely the Act will apply. It is important to remember that the Act applies to organizations and companies with over 20 employees, although those with under this number are expected to abide by the spirit of the provisions.

Broadly, the position under the Act is that unlawful discrimination in employment occurs in the following circumstances:

- when a disabled person is treated less favourably than someone else;
- this treatment is given for a reason relating to that person's disability;
- the reason does not apply to the other person, and
- the treatment cannot be justified.

Such discrimination must not occur in:

- the recruitment and retention of employees;
- promotion and transfers; training and development, and
- the dismissal process.

In addition employers must make reasonable changes to their premises or employment arrangements if these substantially disadvantage a disabled employee, or prospective employee, compared to a non-disabled person.

These provisions sound formidable and very supportive of the situation of many people with MS, and in many respects they may be; however, the detailed interpretation of the provisions of the Act awaits clarification. Many of the provisions of the Act hinge on what a 'substantial' disadvantage to a disabled person is, and what is 'a reasonable' adjustment on the employer's part is. Nevertheless, some examples may help to clarify certain provisions:

- Employers probably cannot justify dismissing disabled employees if they were sometimes off work because of their disability, if the amount of time they take off is what the employers accept as sick leave for other employees.
- Employers cannot justify refusing to promote a person who uses a wheelchair, solely because the person's new workstation is not wheelchair accessible, if by reasonable rearrangement it could be made accessible.
- If an employer requires someone with a particular typing speed, and someone with arthritis of the hands who applies for the job has too slow a speed, the employer has to consider whether any reasonable adjustment could be made. If it could not, the employer can refuse to employ the person.
- Employers have to make any reasonable adjustment needed for disabled people to take part in an interview, to make sure that they would not be at a substantial disadvantage.
- If an employer has not asked about – and the disabled person has not mentioned – any particular needs, then the employer may still have to make some kind of adjustment on finding that the person has a disability, and is at a substantial disadvantage.

'Reasonable' changes to be expected

What 'a reasonable change' is for the benefit of a disabled person depends on:

- how much an alteration will improve the situation for the person;
- how easy it is to make the change;
- the cost of the measure (in terms of finance and disruption);
- the employer's resources;
- financial, or other help, that may be available.

Examples of changes to physical features that may be required are:

- widening doorways;
- changing taps to make them easier to turn;
- altering lighting for people with restricted vision, and
- allocating a particular parking space for a disabled person's car.

Examples of changes to procedures or practices that may be required are:

- altering working hours;
- supplying additional training;
- allocating some duties to another employee;
- allowing absences during working hours for rehabilitation, assessment and treatment;
- providing a reader or interpreter;
- providing supervision;
- acquiring or making changes to equipment;
- modifying procedures for testing or assessment, or
- transferring person to another place of work.

Further information on the provisions of the Act can be obtained from the Disability Discrimination Act Information Line (see Appendix 1). There is also a booklet containing guidance and a code of practice on employment available from the Stationery Office (see Appendix 2).

Exceptions to the Act

Although all permanent, temporary and contract workers are covered, certain organizations or work settings are not covered. These include:

- people in the armed services;
- police officers;
- fire brigade members if they are expected to take part in firefighting;
- Ministry of Defence firefighters
- prison officers and prison custody officers;
- people working on board a ship, aircraft or a hovercraft;
- people who work outside the UK;
- individual franchise holders with less than 20 employees, even if the whole franchise network has more than 20.

If employment levels fluctuate, the Act applies whenever there are 20 employees. As a different kind of exception, there are charities and organizations providing supported employment who can discriminate in favour of disabled people.

Having said that, most employers are understanding and many will go out of their way to support people in similar circumstances, and informing them of your complete circumstances will be beneficial. However, only you can judge how your employer might react to the news of your diagnosis.

13
Finances

This chapter deals with some very complicated issues. This is not only because people's own circumstances are all different, but because the rules and regulations governing eligibility to benefits, pensions and so on are themselves complex and can change frequently. It is very important that, in addition to taking note of the points we make below, you consult other sources of information. Choices that you may make about continuing or leaving work, or about benefits or pensions, may have long-lasting consequences, so it is important to think them through carefully, after seeking impartial advice.

Benefits

Sources of help

The most obvious written source is the *Disability Rights Handbook*. This is updated every April and published by the Disability Alliance (see Appendix 2). This guide is very readable but, unless you are familiar with interpreting legislation, you should still seek advice from other sources.

- The Benefits Agency handles social security payments for the Department of Social Security.
- Your local Citizens Advice is the best source of detailed and impartial information available; there are bureaux across the United Kingdom – the telephone directory will list the address and phone number of your local office, or you can contact the national bureau listed in Appendix 1. They will try to answer questions on almost any issues of concern to you, but will direct you to more appropriate sources of help and advice if you need any.
- Your local authority's welfare rights advisor.
- Welfare advisors at your local branch of the MS Society.
- The Post Office, particularly larger branches and regional offices,

stock a wide range of government forms and leaflets, which are normally prominently displayed. These include leaflets detailing entitlements to health care under the National Health Service, family benefit and disability allowances. Contact addresses and telephone numbers are given for further information in each of these leaflets.

• Your local Employment Service Office (Job Centre) will also stock a range of helpful information, including a pack of employment-related publications that cover most issues related to employment and benefit entitlements. Staff will usually be able to answer specific questions that you have, although you may have to book an appointment in advance.

Stopping work

Benefits available will depend very much on your personal circumstances, the extent of your disability from MS, the nature of your occupation and any health insurance and/or early retirement pensions provision, amongst other factors. This is why you need careful and detailed impartial advice from someone who is able to go through all the aspects of your situation, and point out both the short- and long-term financial consequences of any decision you make.

The first important consideration is whether you are likely to consider a different type of work to that you have been doing, either now or in the future. If you are younger, a considerable way from normal retirement age, this is a crucial issue. Of course the work might be part-time rather than full-time, or involve being self-employed rather than employed. Although MS, as we have said, is very unpredictable, it may be worth discussing your medical outlook with your doctor, particularly regarding your skills and abilities related to the symptoms and any disabilities that you may have now. As a medical assessment of your situation is likely to prove crucial to some of the financial and other benefits you could receive, the role of your doctor – GP or specialist – will be important.

Second, if you have decided that you would like to retire, probably on the grounds of ill-health or disability, then you need to work out how best this can be undertaken. It would be sensible to seek the advice of your Trade Union, if you belong to one, or your professional body, and/or to seek advice from Citizens Advice, before taking any action. How you leave your work – taking early retirement on grounds of ill-health, resigning or being dismissed – also affects the financial benefits for which you may be eligible. Some of these depend on what pension arrangements you might have. You should find out all this from your employer's personnel department or the relevant pensions company. Your employer should help you to retire at the most opportune time for you to gain financially

If you find yourself being peremptorily or unfairly dismissed, you need to seek further advice immediately from your Trade Union, professional body or Citizens Advice. In these circumstances, if you have been employed by your employer for longer than 2 years, you can pursue your case through an industrial tribunal – but again seek advice.

Third, you need to think through carefully the financial consequences of your retirement in the light of your eligibility for a range of benefits. This will depend on many factors. You will need to be realistic about your current and future financial commitments. You may also have to consider your family, as to whether other members of your household are or can be earning, even if you cannot. Even if you have taken early retirement, and thus possibly have an occupational pension, you may still qualify for various means-tested benefits. These may depend not only on your current income, but on your National Insurance Contribution record and your degree of disability. You may be eligible for some or all of these benefits:

- Incapacity Benefit
- Severe Disablement Allowance
- Disability Living Allowance (see *Multiple Sclerosis – the 'at your fingertips' guide* in Appendix 2).

If you do not have an occupational pension you may be eligible for other means-tested benefits, such as:

- Income Support
- Housing Benefit
- Council Tax Benefit.

If you are eligible for Income Support, then you also become eligible for a wide range of other benefits, such as:

- free prescriptions
- free dental treatment
- free school meals for your school-age children.

Help for services and equipment

If you need a particular piece of equipment, a particular service or a holiday, there are funds held by trade unions, professional organizations or charitable bodies for such purposes. Often there is a question of eligibility, but of a different kind than that for the Benefits Agency. You may have to be a current or former member of the organization concerned, or have some other characteristic that gives you entitlement – such as living in a particular area.

The problem is often finding out which organizations you can apply to, for many local charities are small and are not widely advertised. However, there is a *Charities Digest* (your local library should have a copy) which lists many, although not all, sources of funds. Your local library, or Citizens Advice, may be able to give you some sources as well. There is also another directory called *A Guide to Grants for Individuals in Need* which contains a relatively comprehensive list of charities who provide support for individuals with certain eligibility criteria (see Appendix 1). The MS Society can help here too.

Children as carers

There are a number of allowances that may be available, again depending on your eligibility, when you require the support of others for your care. Some benefits are payable to you, and others to those looking after you. There are, as usual, quite complicated eligibility rules about which you will almost certainly need to seek detailed advice. For example, if one of your children is looking after you on virtually a full-time basis (35 hours a week or more), and you have Disability Living Allowance at the middle or higher rate, or Attendance Allowance, then he or she may be eligible for Invalid Care Allowance. You yourself may be able to obtain Attendance Allowance, or the care component of Disability Living Allowance. The criteria for these allowances are very specific, and trying to help your children out might be difficult, without quite a lot of investigation and advice about your and their eligibility from either Citizens Advice or another impartial source of advice about disability.

Mobility

As part of the Disability Living Allowance, it may be possible to claim for the higher or lower rate mobility components to help with additional expenses incurred with your decreased mobility. If you are able to obtain the higher rate component in particular, then it opens the door for a range of other benefits. Both the components are open to people below the age of 65 (or 66 if the disability began at the age of 65). The tests for eligibility for this mobility component are increasingly stringent, and it is not possible to go into them in great detail here; you should seek advice about the criteria and their application to you from the MS Society (see

Appendix 1). As someone with MS, to obtain the higher rate allowance, you will need to demonstrate, in the formal words of the regulations that your 'physical condition as a whole' is such that you are 'unable to walk', or are 'virtually unable to walk', or that 'the exertion required to walk would constitute a danger to [your] life or be likely to lead to a serious deterioration in [your] health'.

There are other criteria under which the higher rate can be claimed but they are unlikely to apply to people with MS. As you can see, the crucial issues in adjudicating any claim for people with MS, apart from when you literally cannot put one step in front of another, are likely to be the meaning of being 'virtually unable to walk', or the relationship of exertion in walking to a possible deterioration in health. In these cases, the assessment process and medical judgements are both critical – the variability of MS does not help. For the lower rate of mobility allowance, the major criterion is not so much whether you are physically able to walk, but whether you require someone most of the time to guide or supervise you, to enable you to walk outdoors.

The *Disability Rights Handbook* published by the Disability Alliance Educational and Research Association (see Appendix 2) has a comprehensive section describing in detail the requirements and procedures for claiming these benefits. You could also telephone or write to the Benefits Agency – which handles such claims for the Department of Social Security – for information on mobility allowances (see Appendix 1). Further help can be obtained through the MS Society's Helpline (the Benefits Advisor) or your local DIAL (Disability Information and Advice Service). If their number is not available in your local telephone book, the Social Services Department of your local council should be able to provide it for you. There are appeal procedures if your claim is turned down. In any case it is very important that you monitor your situation so that, if your mobility decreases through the MS, or indeed through another cause, you claim for the appropriate allowance. Many relevant and useful local addresses can be found in your area telephone book, or the Yellow Pages or Thomson guides.

Wheelchairs

Under the NHS, both hand- and electric-powered wheelchairs are supplied and maintained free of charge for people who are disabled and whose need for a wheelchair is permanent. Although, in principle, any wheelchair can be supplied by the NHS, in practice the decision is made locally, where the circumstances of the individual and local resources will be taken into account. Since April 1996, powered wheelchairs can be provided by the NHS, if you need a wheelchair, cannot walk and cannot propel a wheelchair yourself. Again local decisions are made about provision of such wheelchairs, although it is anticipated that local decisions will fit with the broader national criteria. These include being able to handle the wheelchair safely, and being able to benefit from an improved quality of life in a wheelchair. If you already have a wheelchair, move to new area and do not meet the local criteria in that area, you can still keep your wheelchair – unless there are clinical reasons for withdrawing it. Attendant-controlled powered wheelchairs can also be issued where it is difficult for the person to be pushed outdoors – if the area is very hilly, if the person is heavy, or the attendant is elderly and unable to push a wheelchair manually.

There are voucher schemes operated by NHS Trusts whereby people can contribute towards the costs of a more expensive wheelchair than a Trust would provide. Schemes either give responsibility to the Trust for repair and maintenance of the wheelchair, or allow you to take responsibility yourself. You may not be able to use this scheme to obtain a powered wheelchair, but it may be possible to use the Motability Scheme to obtain such a wheelchair. Wheelchairs, pavement vehicles (usually electrically operated wheelchairs or scooters), crutches and walking frames are exempt from VAT.

The MS Society branches and HQ can offer advice on financial help for wheelchairs or even provide one in some cases.

Driving

There are a number of benefits for which you may be eligible as a driver. If you receive the higher rate mobility allowance you will be allowed to claim exemption from vehicle excise duty (road tax) on one vehicle. This exemption is given on condition that the vehicle is used 'solely for the purposes of the disabled person', so care must be taken as to the use of the vehicle. Nevertheless, it is likely that some commonsense latitude will be given.

If you have the higher rate mobility allowance, you will be automatically eligible for the Blue Badge, which gives parking privileges, and also for access to the Motability Scheme (see below). You will also get VAT exemption on adaptations to make your car suitable for driving by you, as well as exemption on the repair, maintenance or replacement of these adaptations.

Note that the mobility allowance does not count as income for these purposes. Furthermore arrears will not count as capital for means-tested benefits for up to 1 year after they are paid.

Insurance

Telling your insurance company

In the case of health insurance, life assurance or endowment policies associated with a mortgage, you must tell the company that you have MS. Such information may also be required for car insurance purposes in order to ensure that any future claim you make will not be denied, on the grounds that you had not told the company about MS. As you will probably be aware, insurance application forms generally have a 'catch-all' request that you provide 'any information that you feel may be relevant', or a similar wording. What this means is that, if you have failed to provide information that the insurance company – not just yourself – feels is relevant to a claim that you may make at a later date, then the claim could be invalidated and it will not be met. In this case the burden is on you, as the insured or the applicant, to disclose information relevant to any future claim, and ensure that the full facts are given when the insurance is first taken out.

For existing policies, you are obliged to give all details of any changes in your circumstances, whenever your insurance is renewed. However, so long as the changes in circumstances (e.g. a diagnosis of MS) occurred after you took out the policy, there should – in principle – be no substantial change in the terms of your insurance, although the company may make enquiries as to whether in fact you did know about the MS when taking out that insurance.

Almost all health insurance policies carry exclusions for 'pre-existing conditions' which is taken to mean any condition of which there was significant evidence before insurance commenced. In the case of a condition such as MS, this would include any tests or examinations that you have had for MS, including all those that you underwent before diagnosis. It is wise to be as accurate and as detailed as possible to give as few grounds as you can for exclusion at a later date. It is worth noting that few insurance companies will refuse to insure you, although most will charge higher premiums when there is a reasonable cause to expect a higher risk of claims.

Do be careful to read the terms of any attractive policy that guarantees acceptance and has fixed premiums. The maximum payout and range of exclusions may seriously limit the value of the cover, and a 'no questions asked, no medicals' policy can still exclude claims where the insured failed to provide information when the cover was taken out.

New policies and renewals

Although insurance companies can, and sometimes do refuse to insure people with conditions like MS, their usual response is to load the premiums according to the risks they estimate of you making a claim. Although these risks are calculated (or should be) on the basis of what are called 'actuarial tables', which provide information on how long people of certain ages, genders, or with certain conditions live, or are likely at any rate not to make a claim, sometimes insurance companies may load premiums even further if they do not want a particular kind of business. You may find quite big differences between insurance companies in the way they respond to information about MS. More recently there has developed what might be described as a 'niche' insurance market which is beginning to specialize in people with disabilities and certain kinds of medical condition; you might find this more supportive. There are also now life policies, particularly for older people over 50, that guarantee acceptance, and pay out fixed sums after 2 years without a medical examination or other questions needed. These may seem like a good idea, and indeed, they can provide additional money for your family if you die. However, generally, the benefits are fixed amounts of money so that, if you do live a long time, you find yourself paying more in premiums than would be returned in benefits if you die.

On health – as opposed to life – insurance you may find some difficulty getting a new policy, or it may contain key exclusions, related to some of the more common medical complications of MS. A company may also be concerned about another issue, which is whether you will be able to continue to pay the premiums, if they are substantial, and they feel that there is a risk that you may not be able to continue in employment. This seems to be very unfair, but insurance companies are essentially commercial concerns, and thus their bottom line is the balance between premium income and future claims.

The moral is that in all cases you need to seek impartial advice, to shop around, and to consider very carefully any conditions or exclusions to policies – in short you must read the small print!

Mortgages

Mortgage lenders take many factors into account, including your savings, your income and the security of your employment, and of course how much you may wish to borrow. However, the key factor will be the company's estimation of how likely you will be able to continue paying for your mortgage until its term is complete. In this respect, different companies may take a different view of the future, partly depending on whether they feel you will be able to keep in employment for the term of the mortgage. Some may take a more pessimistic view than others of the progress and effects of your MS, so it is important that you shop around, as with other major financial transactions.

Healthcare finance

Prescriptions

Unfortunately you are not entitled to free prescriptions just because you have MS – it is not yet included as one of the relatively few diseases or conditions for which free prescriptions are available. However, prescriptions are free if you are aged under 16 or in full-time education and aged under 19; if you are aged over 60; or if you are either pregnant, or have had a baby within the last 12 months. In these cases you need only to sign the appropriate section of the prescription form. Prescriptions are also free when you are receiving many forms of state benefit and this may also apply to your partner or dependent children.

If you or your partner are on state benefits (specifically Income Support, Jobseeker's Allowance, Family Credit, or Disability Working Allowance), you can also claim free prescriptions. Some prescriptions are also free for people receiving hospital care or diagnosed with very specific medical conditions not including MS itself, but including some of its possible complications such as genitourinary infections. There are also a number of other specific circumstances in which free prescriptions may be available, and these need to be checked out with your local Social Security Office.

In some of these circumstances you will require a completed HC1, HC2 or HC3 form and certificate number. You can obtain the form from a Social Security office, NHS hospital, dentist or doctor.

Even if you are not entitled to free prescriptions, you can save money if you need more than five items in 4 months or more than 14 items in 12 months by using a pre-payment certificate. You will need to get an application form FP95 from a Post Office or pharmacy.

Eye and dental care costs

In addition to free prescriptions, most of the categories of entitlement listed above also entitle you to NHS (not private) dental care, eye tests and glasses or contact lenses. Necessary costs of travel to hospital for NHS treatment include the cost of travel for a partner or helper if you are unable to travel alone.

Given the high costs of prescription, eye care and dental treatment, it is well worth exercising your claim to whatever qualifying benefits you are entitled, in order then to have these free treatments, even if you feel the qualifying benefit itself is of relatively little value to you.

There is information about finance and caring in the *Respite and residential care* section in Chapter 15.

Managing finances

Power of Attorney

You may, at some point, feel the need for someone to take over your financial arrangements. If so, you will almost certainly need good legal advice, perhaps at first from Citizens Advice if you have not already got a good solicitor. Because this situations tends to happen when you get older, and some good documentation is available from Age Concern, especially their Factsheet Number 22: *Legal Arrangements for Managing Financial Affairs*. There are two versions, one for England and Wales and the other for Scotland. Age Concern offices will have these available (see Appendix 1 for their address).

There are a range of options that a relative (or friend) might consider, from very limited permissions to deal with specific issues, to more all-embracing powers, including what is called an Enduring Power of Attorney, which enables someone to act virtually in all respects on your behalf in financial matters. A special form is necessary for a Power of Attorney, which gives someone the right to act for you; you will need to sign it, as will your relative and a witness – usually not a family member, but someone who is independent. If, after signing, you become incapable of understanding the situation, then your relative will need to apply to the Court of Protection (part of the Supreme Court) for the Power of Attorney to be recognized, so that he or she can continue to act without your formal consent. If you cannot understand the situation and a Power of Attorney has not been obtained, your relative will have to apply to the Court of Protection (in England) requesting it to act as the 'Receiver' of your affairs.

The complex procedures are designed to ensure that a decision to take over someone else's financial affairs is not taken lightly. It does mean that it is far easier, and less costly, to try and deal with this problem at an early stage, when it can be done with the understanding and agreement of all parties.

By the way, it is also important to make your Will, if you have not already done so; it becomes a complex area of law when a person has failed to make a Will, and subsequently interpretations have to be made of their wishes or intentions.

Financially planning for a child when you have MS

If you have not yet written a Will, you ought to do so. Consider the nature of your estate (including your house if you own one), and how best to ensure that the part of it you wish to use for your child is available, with the least taxation as is legally possible on your death. Even if you have made a Will, you may need to ensure that the process of passing on resources is as tax efficient as possible. You will almost certainly need to seek legal and financial advice. If you do not already have a solicitor, get advice first at Citizens Advice in your area.

Another issue is whether it is sensible to transfer some of your assets at an earlier stage than your death to your child. This may have some long-term tax advantages. On the other hand it may reduce the eligibility of your child for certain state benefits both currently and in the future.

Also, another thing to consider is whether your child is likely to be able to manage his or her own finances if you die, and you might need some arrangement whereby someone can manage the financial affairs – in the child's interests, of course. There are a number of formal ways in which this can be organized – through the setting up of a Trust with your child as a beneficiary, for example. These considerations are invariably complex and need a detailed knowledge of the relevant legal situation; you need sound judgement about the long-term as well as the short-term financial consequences of the chosen course of action. It would be unwise to make major decisions on these issues without impartial advice.

14
Housing and home adaptations

Housing issues can become particularly difficult for people with MS and their families. This may be because funds to support your existing accommodation as you have become used to it become less through having to work part-time or indeed having to give up work altogether. Of course, other difficulties, especially related to decreasing mobility, may mean that your existing accommodation, or a significant part of it, could become harder and harder to manage without adaptation.

Most people with MS will wish to stay in their own homes. Factors affecting any decisions to stay or move will include your income, how easy the home is to adapt, and what kinds of services are available from the local Social Services and Housing Departments.

Getting help for housing adaptations

One of the issues that may be a major consideration to someone with MS as well as those living with them, is the need – at some point – to consider adaptations to their home to ensure that everybody can live comfortably and easily in it. A variety of adaptations may prove necessary, although each individual person may well require a different pattern of such adaptations. They are likely to range from installation of stairlifts, to adaptations to living rooms, bedrooms, kitchens, bathrooms and toilets, to making access easier both within the property, as well as into and out of it. Obviously many possible adaptations will not only depend on your own disabilities, but also on the nature and state of the property that you are currently living in.

If you consider that you cannot continue to live in your current house without changes to the accommodation, there is a grant called the Disabled Facilities Grant (DFG) for which you may be eligible. This is available for owner occupiers, private and housing association tenants, and landlords, and is given by the department of the local council responsible for housing. The person with MS need not personally make an application, for others can do this for them, although they have to demonstrate their right to do so. The maximum mandatory amount that can be awarded is £20,000, although local authorities have discretion to award more than this.

Mandatory and discretionary awards are given for different purposes. Mandatory grants can be used to:

- facilitate access to and from the property concerned;
- make the property safe for those living in it;
- ensure the disabled person can access the principal family room;
- adapt the kitchen to enable the cooking and preparation of food independently;
- provide access to a room used for sleeping;
- provide or improve access to the toilet, wash basin, bath (and/or shower);
- improve or provide a heating system in the property for the disabled person;
- adapt heating, lighting or power controls to make them easier to use;
- improve access and movement around the home to enable a disabled occupant to care for another person who normally lives with them.

Discretionary awards can be used to adapt the property to make it more suitable for the accommodation, welfare or employment of the disabled occupant.

There is a means test – both of the disabled person and what are called 'relevant persons' – for this Disability Facilities Grant, and you might have to contribute to the cost, depending on your financial situation. For most people with MS, the relevant person will be their spouse/partner – in addition to themselves, or a parent(s) if the person is under 18. The financial assessments are quite complicated and take into account savings (above £5000), as well as weekly income, set against an assessment of needs as recognized by allowances that the person with MS may have. RADAR has produced an information pack entitled *Meeting the Cost of Adaptations* which you may find helpful.

If you feel that you cannot afford what the local authority indicates you should contribute, then you can ask the Social Services department to make a 'top up' payment or loan. The department can also help with top-up funding for a DFG if the cost is above £20,000 and the council housing department is only giving a grant up to the £20,000 limit for mandatory Disability Facilities Grants. Such (albeit discretionary) support has been important to many disabled people who could not obtain full funding for adaptations through their Disability Facilities Grant.

Note that certain adaptations are zero rated for VAT purposes, i.e. the builder will not charge you 17.5% VAT on top of the bill for certain jobs, saving you about a sixth of the bill. Such zero rating will normally include the construction of ramps, widening of doorways and passages to facilitate access by a disabled person; installation of a lift between floors to facilitate access, including maintenance, repair and restoration of decorations, and works to bathrooms and toilets to facilitate use and access by the disabled occupant and any goods supplied in connection with this.

Overall, in deciding whether to make an award, the housing department of the local authority will consider, in consultation with social services, whether the works are necessary and appropriate to the needs of a disabled person. They will also consider whether the adaptations are reasonable and practicable taking into account the age and condition of the property. This might lead to alternative possibilities being considered. These might include urging the disabled occupant to seek a renovation grant to make the property fit, considering whether a reduced level of adaptations to the property would be feasible, and finally considering with the disabled person the option of re-housing. One organization offering help in relation to agencies who can assist you on these issues is Care and Repair (address in Appendix 1).

Getting help for housing repairs

If you are living in an older property, or even if you are not, there may well be an issue about the property needing repairs. As we have seen in the section above, the possibility of financial support of adaptations to your property might well be linked, amongst other things, to its current state of repair.

If you are not able to pay for repairs yourself, you may be able to get a renovation grant from the council. This is likely to be the case if your home needs extensive repair or improvement work, or if you lack a basic facility such as an indoor toilet or a bath or shower. Home owners and some tenants, although not council tenants, can apply for a renovation grant. You should not assume that you will automatically receive a grant, as they are awarded at the discretion of the Local Authority. The grant is subject to a means test, which assesses how much you will have to contribute towards the cost of works. You will have to contact your local Housing Department for further information and an application form.

Grants of up to £2000 can be made, or up to £4000 for separate applications for housing repairs in any 3 years. Home repair assistance is a discretionary grant. The main purpose for which the grant is available is smaller-scale, but still essential, repairs or adaptations. This grant is open to home owners and tenants of private landlords and housing associations. Home repair assistance need not involve an occupational therapist assessment or a means test, although practices vary from one area to another. It is important that applicants ask the council for guidelines on who has priority for the grant in their area before they start putting information together for the application.

Re-housing

It may be a good idea to look at whether other housing might be better for you. This may well depend on your finances, and on whether you own or rent your current home. Even if you do own your own home, you could still discuss the situation with the Housing Department of your local authority; also, housing associations operating locally may have a special interest in people with disabilities.

The Housing Department has a responsibility for considering people's housing problems whether or not they own their own homes. However, how far you get in your request will depend on several factors, including the severity of your problems, housing resources available locally, your financial situation, the demand for the type of housing you may wish to apply for, and any particular local conditions (financial or otherwise) attached to local authority re-housing.

You can apply to go on the housing register of your Local Authority (which often used to be called the waiting list). This is the main route to permanent housing. It is important that, whatever your circumstances, you go on the housing register if you require permanent accommodation.

For the register, you will be asked to provide basic details such as your name, the number of people in your household and whether they are under 10 years of age or over 60 years old, and your address. Further information that may be held on the register could include details of any disability involved and specific housing requirements.

After the council has agreed that you are eligible to go on the housing register, your re-housing priority will be decided. The council will look at your circumstances, your present accommodation, and what kind of accommodation you require, using the information that you give them on the application form and medical form to decide your priority. Under the Housing Act 1996, the council has to give reasonable preference for re-housing to the following people:

- people occupying unsanitary or overcrowded, or otherwise living in unsatisfactory, housing conditions;
- people occupying housing accommodation that is temporarily occupied on insecure terms;
- families with dependent children;
- households consisting of or including someone who is expecting a child;
- households consisting of or including someone with a particular need for settled accommodation on welfare on medical grounds;
- households whose social or economic circumstances are such that they have difficulty in securing settled accommodation.

Additional preference is given where a member of the household has a particular need for settled accommodation on welfare or medical grounds and who cannot reasonably be expected to find settled accommodation themselves in the near future. This can include those who are particularly vulnerable as a result of old age, physical or mental illness, and/because of a learning or physical disability. If a person in this situation could live independently with the necessary support, but could not be expected to secure accommodation on their own initiative, then they should get additional preference for re-housing.

The main categories affecting people with a disability as a result of MS are the first and fifth bullets above. The first category could be relevant if you are a disabled person living in inaccessible housing. This could constitute unsatisfactory housing conditions. The fifth category is for people who need settled (i.e. long-term) accommodation on welfare or medical grounds. When assessing medical grounds, the council will be expected to take into account advice from medical professionals. Guidance from the Government to local councils make it clear that this fifth category is designed to apply to disabled people.

The council may involve Social Services and Health Authorities in assessing whether a household has a particular need for long-term settled accommodation. You can receive reasonable preference for re-housing under more than one category, so you can 'build up' your priority for re-housing. For example, you could have priority for re-housing because of your disability as well as because you have dependent children.

If you are seeking to move either to another house as an owner-occupier, or into the privately rented sector, you will probably realize that there is no central register, or one key source of information, on which properties are 'disability friendly'. Although recent legislation has required all new houses being built to be more disability friendly than they were, clearly there is enormous variety amongst the existing housing stock in terms of its suitability for people with mobility or other difficulties.

Finding accessible housing can be difficult. Estate agents do not routinely inspect properties for their accessibility. In order to avoid wasted visits to estate agents or letting agencies, you should write to any in your chosen area setting out briefly the basic requirements you are looking for. Try to make them simple and straightforward and do not necessarily expect them to understand what, for example, a wheelchair user would require. Always be aware of the possibility of adapting a property.

It is also worth looking in the disability newspapers and local disability newsletters for advertisements from disabled people selling or renting out properties. You could also consider placing an advertisement in one of these asking if anyone has a suitable property for sale or rent. Contact your local disability organization to see if they know of suitable properties in the area, or whether they let you put up an advert in their offices or centre. There may also be a Disabled Persons' Housing Service, Disabled Persons' Accommodation Agency or Register in your chosen area. These not-for-profit organizations will be able to help you find suitable property to buy or rent.

Sheltered housing

Sheltered housing is accommodation specially built for people who may need some additional supervision or support to that normally available, but who still wish to maintain a substantial degree of independence. There are various forms of supervision and support: some accommodation just has a warden on site who can be contacted in an emergency; other sheltered housing is relatively high dependency where staff assist with meals and personal care, but where there is still some privacy and independence.

Providers of such accommodation include local authorities, housing associations and private companies, or sometimes a combination of one or more of these. Usually the Housing Department of your local authority will be able to give you information on providers of such housing in your area.

15
Care

The variety of care is very substantial. In fact the word 'care' is used in such a range of ways that, to a degree, it has lost much of its original and particular meaning. In this chapter we focus on 'care' in the sense of the formal provision of services by mainly statutory health or social care bodies for people with MS and their families. The degree to which such services constitute individual 'care' as considered for people with MS and their families is a matter of (their) judgement. Indeed the perennial issue for people with MS is the degree to which health care and social care services can meet both the diversity and scale of their care needs.

Care in the community

'Community care' is the general name given to services provided to help people with an illness or disability to continue to live in their own homes. At the same time, there has been an associated policy to provide sheltered housing and residential and nursing homes in 'the community' for such people who cannot continue to live in their own home.

The Community Care Act (1992) provides the framework for community care. This Act gives Social Services Departments the responsibility to assess people's needs through a 'needs assessment', and to provide, or to purchase from others, a range of services to meet those needs. The assumption behind the provision of these services is that they will enable the person to remain in their own homes as long as possible.

'Community care' covers a wide range of services that are designed to support people in their own homes – but the nature and type of these services varies considerably from area to area. As might be expected, local financial constraints have a major effect on what services are provided, and indeed when a judgement may be made that it is no longer viable to support someone at home. It is important to note that local authorities (through their Social Services Departments) are not obliged to continue to support someone at home, if this would cost more than moving them to a residential or nursing home – although sometimes they may continue to provide services for the person at home. This issue, amongst several other major issues, has been – and indeed still is – the subject of legal argument as to the exact obligations of local authorities under the Community Care Act.

Health services versus social services

In addition there can be problems in 'community care' arising from the role of health services in relation to social services. Some community-based services, such as nursing help or physiotherapy, are obtained through the NHS (via your GP or hospital specialist), whilst others, such as home help or meals on wheels, are obtained via social services (usually through a needs assessment under the Community Care Act). However, a number of practical difficulties have arisen as to when a service is a 'health' service, when it is a 'social' service, and, most importantly, who (the NHS or local authorities) should pay for it. Although there has been a series of firm government attempts to produce a cooperative environment between health and social services, people with MS may still find that they are in an uncomfortable position between two major service suppliers. Nevertheless, if you feel that you are in need of community service support, you must ask for a Social Services needs assessment.

Community health services are now being increasingly provided through a new range of organizations called 'Primary Health Care Trusts'. Although such Trusts are not yet established in all areas of the UK, their numbers are increasing rapidly. It has been government policy that priority must be given to primary health and community-based care, whereas previously the focus was much more on hospital care. In a number of cases 'Community Health Care Trusts', which had combined the provision of both hospital and community-based care, are now giving way to Trusts based entirely on primary and community are. The services provided through the community/primary care-based trusts include district nurses, health visitors, community psychiatric and mental health nurses, psychologists, physiotherapists, occupational therapists, speech and language therapists, dietitians and chiropodists. There may also be specific services for incontinence, cardiac care, mastectomy and colostomy. In some areas there are specific MS nurses who act in a wide-ranging role. Most of these services are obtained through your GP or practice nurse, but in some areas they may still be organized through hospitals.

There are a range of collaborative arrangements between Community Health Services. In some places the collaboration works well and in others less well. Increasingly formal collaborative arrangements are being set up, with the Social Services care manager acting as the main liaison between the person with MS and the service providers. However, as the management structures, funding sources and professional tasks of Social Services and Community Health Services are different, the link between the two may not always work well – even though they both emphasize their service to the person with MS.

Needs assessments

A needs assessment is organized by Social Services when they think that someone may need community services. The assessment is usually carried out either by a social worker or an occupational therapist; you will have to complete a questionnaire. The views of the GP, other professional staff and your carer, if you have one, will be taken into account.

Care managers

A 'care manager' will be appointed, if you are granted services, to manage a 'care plan' – this will state the nature, type and frequency of community services you may receive.

This plan will be monitored and appropriate changes made to it as your situation changes. The care manager will be the main line of communication to the Social Services Department, and the main means through whom any problems can be remedied or resolved. A good care manager will be supportive and helpful.

Services available

Financial constraints and the differential availability of services locally may mean that relatively few are available for any one person. The list in the box overleaf shows (again in principle!) the kinds of services that might be made available, depending on the results of the needs assessment, local resources available, and the organization of health, social service and voluntary sector cooperation.

Carers needs

If you have a carer, and you share the house with that person, then he or she can request their own needs assessment. This is not a check as to whether they are 'good' at caring; it is to check whether they are getting the support needed to carry on caring.

Carers' needs assessments are carried out by Social Services Departments under the arrangements in the Carers (Recognition and Services) Act (1995). Such a needs assessment can be considered only in conjunction with your own needs assessment.

Social Services are not under any legal obligation to provide help for carers, but an assessment may put you in a stronger position to argue for more support or, for example, respite care.

The Carers National Association (Carers UK) has a helpline which provides advice on carers' needs assessments. It publishes helpful booklets on caring aspects (see Appendix 1).

SERVICES AVAILABLE

In your home

- adaptations of various kinds
- alarm systems
- various benefits
- equipment
- help from Good Neighbour or Care Attendant schemes
- home helps or carers
- home visits from various professionals
- homemaker schemes (someone to look after your home if your carer temporarily cannot)
- home library service
- laundry service
- meals on wheels
- odd job schemes (practical help for odd jobs in the home)
- recreational facilities (TV and radio)
- sitting in or sleeping in services (allowing a carer a day or night away)
- social work support
- telephone services

Outside the home

- day centres
- day hospital care
- education work centres
- holiday/short-term care
- medical escort service (to get to hospital)
- respite or short-stay care

Medical services

- occupational therapy
- physiotherapy
- speech and language therapy
- general rehabilitation

Disagreeing with the assessment

There are many complicated (and controversial) issues regarding needs assessments, and particularly in the balance between physical capacity to undertake tasks, and emotional, or psychological reasons that may make this difficult. This can be a particular problem in the area of personal care, where there may be strong social, emotional or personal inhibitions in one family member undertaking toileting or bathing for another – especially where they are of opposite genders, or of different generations. In the needs assessment itself, one Social Services Department (or one social worker) may feel that 'need' (for other services) is not present, and that you are physically capable of undertaking the task, even though you may find it personally very difficult, or damaging to your relationship with your partner . Of course, local financial constraints may also mean that very stringent definitions of 'need' rule out a more sensitive approach to such issues. An appeal may be necessary against such a needs assessment if you feel strongly about it.

Appeals

If you do not agree with the needs assessment or with the care plan you have been given, the first course of action is to contact your care manager – usually an occupational therapist or social worker, to discuss your concerns in order to try and resolve them. If you are still not satisfied, you should write formally to the Director of Social Services (or the Complaints Officer if the Social Services Department has one) and ask for it to be registered as a formal complaint. You may ask someone else to help you write the letter. Someone (not the person who undertook the original needs assessment or devised the care plan) will investigate your complaint and you must receive a reply within 28 days from the authority's receipt of your formal complaint. If you are not satisfied with the authority's reply, you can ask for your complaint to be heard by a review panel within 28 days of the date when you received that reply. You can be accompanied by someone to support you at the hearing of the panel, and the local authority must give its response to the findings of the review panel within 28 days. This procedure has been used with increasing frequency to try and clarify the basis on which community care services are provided, with a number of disputed cases going on to the High Court for final resolution.

Home helps versus home care workers

It is not always clear exactly what the distinction is, and there may be some overlap. However, in general a home help undertakes cleaning duties, whereas home care workers concentrate on personal care, and may be forbidden to undertake any cleaning.

Respite and residential care

When someone with MS is significantly disabled in terms of the everyday tasks that they can perform, it is not always possible for them to remain in a home setting continuously – even with help from family, friends and the health and social services. Other options may have to be considered; these might include a temporary and occasional break through being cared for elsewhere, to longer term and more permanent care outside the home. People have very different views about these situations, and how to manage them. They are not often easy to discuss, let alone act upon. This is not least because such options almost always involve the separation of the person with MS, from their partner or other family members, and this adds to the anxieties and concerns of all parties to the discussions.

Respite care

Respite care is often thought of as a need for a break from partners, not just from their care. This need not be the case at all, and a break is needed purely from the tasks of actual caring. However, it is expensive, and practically more complicated to provide respite care for two people rather than one. There are therefore currently very few places for couples in respite or short-term residential care when one partner has MS, and you will be fortunate if you find such a facility. Given the importance of maintaining a good relationship with your partner, you could lobby your local authority about this problem and/or discuss it with the welfare officer of the local branch of the MS Society.

Residential care

There are several benefits that may well be affected if you go into permanent residential care outside your home. These are Disability Living Allowance, Attendance Allowance, Income Support and Income Job-Seekers Allowance, Housing Benefit, Council Tax Benefit, together with one or two benefits targeted on special groups of people. The rules governing exactly how these benefits are affected are different in each case, so you should seek advice, initially from Citizens Advice, before you make any decision about going into residential care.

Costs

Unless you negotiate independently for residential care, and then pay yourself, under the NHS and Community Care Act 1990 local authorities are empowered to charge you for the cost of providing such care, whether they provide it themselves or use an independent home. The local authority fixes a standard rate for the cost of its own accommodation, or bases it on what it is charged in providing a place in an independent home. If you cannot pay the appropriate rate then the local authority will assess your ability to pay and, on the basis of the criteria, decide what to charge. It is important to note that the assessment would be of your partner's financial status alone, not of your joint status, if you have a partner. Although a local authority can approach a spouse and ask for a 'reasonable' contribution to the support of the resident, there is no formal definition as to what is reasonable – and an unmarried partner has no obligation in this respect.

The criteria by which liability to pay some or all of the costs of residential care are assessed are rather complex. They will consist of investigating your financial status, in terms of both capital and income, and then making certain kinds of allowances for personal expenses. It is very important that, if you are considering residential care, you should seek advice about the costs for which you would be liable well before you enter into any agreement. Citizens Advice should be able to help you in this respect, and you may well have a local disability information service which can also assist you.

16
Leisure, sport and holidays

Although MS itself may cause some problems from time to time, and interrupt your life more than you might like, it is important to keep your leisure activities going as much as you can, not least because many of these will have given you a great deal of enjoyment in the past. They will also enable you to keep in touch with old friends, and make new ones. Indeed, leisure, sport and holidays may also enable you to place MS far more in perspective.

Compared to a few years ago, there are a rapidly increasing number of opportunities for leisure, sport and holidays for people with MS with a range of disabilities.

General information on leisure activities and hobbies

In many local areas there is a wide variety of sources of information about the availability of, and support for, leisure and recreational activities. Many general local facilities, such as swimming pools, sports centres, adult education colleges, cinemas, theatres and so on, have facilities for disabled people, and improvements to access and facilities are developing all the time. There is often an active local group dedicated to your particular interest. The service concerned or the centre in which the activity takes place should be able to give you the details – just give them a ring or visit them and tell them exactly what you require. Your local disability group, local social services or local library should also be able to provide you with information.

Do not be put off if your own particular interests appear not to be provided for at local day centres or at adult education evening classes. This may merely be the result of a perceived lack of demand, and almost any subject can be covered by an evening class when that need is demonstrated. Push for what you are interested in, use the relevant national contact organization to give you back-up and information if necessary, and get other local people involved.

Local authorities are empowered under the Chronically Sick & Disabled Persons Act 1970 to help disabled people to enjoy a wide range of recreational activities. For instance, they may help people obtain a radio, television or similar leisure facility, and go on holiday. They may also provide lectures, games, outings and many other leisure pursuits, including social and youth clubs, and may help with travel to and from home. These recreational activities are covered under Section 2 of the 1970 Act. Contact your social service department to ask for an assessment of your need for any such activity and to see if you fit the local eligibility criteria.

Some local authorities also operate a travelling library service, which will call regularly at the homes of those who are unable to visit libraries. The arrangements for all local authority services differ considerably from area to area but it is certainly worth making enquiries via your social services.

The PLANET (Play Leisure Advice Network) is a national information resource on all aspects of play and leisure for disabled people, and will be able to locate the headquarters of organizations specific to your leisure and hobby interests. These groups in their turn will be able to give you local contact details if they have branches or other contacts (see Appendix 1 for contact details).

In addition to information that you can obtain through the MS Society, you may well find other groups offer help or support with a good knowledge of any disabilities that you might have, such as PHAB clubs which are for anyone with and without a disability. There are numerous PHAB clubs around the UK, offering varied programmes of social activities (see Appendix 1 for contact details).

Sport

You should try keep as active as possible – especially if your mobility is affected. It is even more important that you try and exercise regularly to try and keep your muscles and joints working as well as you can (see Chapter 8). A very active sport may not be possible for all people with the disease, but activities like swimming are possible for many. People also enjoy tennis, squash, badminton, bowls, walking and snooker.

The key thing is to make a judgement about how you actually feel (rather than what you might fear or worry about!) during and after an activity or sport. Different people with MS seem to have somewhat different reactions to activity; for example, some have a problem after getting very hot. If you do have concerns about particular sports, do consult your doctor and/or physiotherapist.

There are specialist facilities for an increasing number of sports and organizations offering advice and support. There are many organizations specifically assisting disabled people's interests in sport and leisure. Disability Sport England develops and coordinates sporting opportunities for disabled people. It has details of organizations connected to specific sports, for example, the British Association of Cricketers with Disabilities and the National Co-ordinating Committee for Swimming For People with Disabilities. In Wales there is also the Federation of Sports Associations for the Disabled in Wales, in Northern Ireland the British Sports Association for the Disabled – Northern Ireland; and in Scotland the Scottish Sports Association for People with a Disability (SSAD).

You may find that you need some additional or specialist equipment to enable you to gain most from your chosen sport. Apart from items commonly used in the chosen sport and easily commercially available, there is a range of sport and leisure equipment produced by individuals, clubs and companies to overcome any particular difficulties you may face. If you need specialized equipment, it is likely that the organization connected to the sport or hobby (see above) will be able to give you practical advice based on personal experience. If the required item is not commercially available you may find REMAP of help. REMAP is a voluntary organization with a network of panels specializing in adapting or designing and making one-off items of equipment for disabled individuals (see Appendix 1 for details).

Gardening

There are many ways you can continue gardening, which can give so much pleasure, and many other people without MS find that they have to adapt the kind of gardening they do, either when their mobility or flexibility changes, or when they get older. Raised flower or vegetable beds help those with mobility problems, or those who are in wheelchairs, to continue gardening. Container-based gardening inside or outside is another possibility. In addition there are special aids and equipment.

The principles of gardening are obviously just the same whether someone has MS or not, but the tools and methods of working may need consideration. It is usually unnecessary to buy a lot of new tools – first consider what tasks you need to carry out, assess your usage of the tools you already have, and consider any adaptations that could be made to make them work to your benefit (such as adding longer handles). With careful planning, the work required in the garden can be reduced.

There are many books on plants that require less maintenance, on making gardening easier, and on accessible garden design. There are several books you can use to help you (see Appendix 2 for details).

Another organization that promotes horticulture for people with disabilities is Horticulture for All. The Gardens for Disabled Trust raises money to help those who are disabled take an active interest in gardening, and gives advice to those who wish to adapt their gardens (see Appendix 1).

Day trips out

Managers of theatres, cinemas or concert halls have generally been slow to understand and provide for the needs of people with disabilities. However, the situation is changing rapidly and people are more aware of the importance of disabled customers; negative publicity about access and other problems has helped push this along. Whilst many venues are more prepared for people with disabilities, it is a still a good idea to contact the management before you go, to explain your situation and what you will need. Some seats, or positions for wheelchairs, may be better than others, and notifying the venue in advance should ensure that your needs are better catered for. You may also find that certain performances (for example, matinées) are less crowded than others.

Provision for people with disabilities at cinemas has improved enormously in the last few years. There are still some problems for disabled cinema-goers, however, owing to the number of older 1930's cinemas which have been converted into several screens. The 'main' screen is often in the circle of the old cinema and accessed only by several steps. However, a good number of ground-floor screens have wheelchair spaces with flat access, or via a few steps, possibly through a side exit.

An increasing number of cinemas are using automatic computerized booking systems via the phone, where you can pay for your ticket by credit card and simply collect it on arrival. Some have an enquiry method for disabled patrons that puts you through to the management to make necessary arrangements. The larger cinemas have facilities available such as seats that provide additional leg room. To find out about the facilities for disabled patrons, contact the cinema showing your choice of film direct and ask for details.

As far as theatres go, many of the larger venues now have adapted toilets and facilities. In some theatres, it may be necessary for the occupant of a wheelchair to be able to transfer into an aisle seat, with the wheelchair stowed elsewhere. In other theatres, seats can be removed with advance notice to make way for a wheelchair, while in others there are specific seat-less areas where a wheelchair user will be asked to sit. If you need assistance or a specific seat as an ambulant or visually impaired disabled person, or indeed for any disability, then do ask in advance. Usually the easiest access to seats will be on the same level as any wheelchair spaces, and/or you could ask for a seat at the end of a row if this is helpful.

For other popular venues such as museums, galleries or arts centres, if you are unsure about access and facilities, contact the place concerned and ask in advance of your visit. Both access and the presentation of exhibits have been improved to suit disabled visitors, and facilities, such as catering and the provision of toilets, have been upgraded as well. Some major museums and galleries are large, making it difficult to walk or wheel all the way round in a single visit. Like most visitors, you may prefer to look at a museum/gallery map before or when you arrive, so you can select some of the things of greatest interest and plan the easiest route round. Some places will have on-site wheelchairs to borrow, but check and book these in advance if they are going to be a necessity. Ask about any entrance charges – most are free.

Some arts centres are housed in modern, purpose-built buildings; others are based in old buildings such as Victorian town halls and churches that have been adapted for the purpose. Accessibility varies, but efforts have been made in recent years to cater better for disabled visitors. Many arts venues have multiple functions, and may include a cinema, theatre, concert hall, and an exhibition area. If you are in London, you may find it practical as well as interesting to visit a site or complex that has a number of such accessible possibilities within easy reach of each other, such as the South Bank or the Barbican centre.

If you are going to a theatre, cinema or other venue in London, you could contact the London arts access information service, Artsline. As well as providing a telephone information line, Artsline has available an access guide to theatres in London called *Open Door* and a booklet entitled *Disabled Access Guide to London's West End Theatres* (see Appendices 1 and 2).

You should also check to see whether there are any services giving similar information in your area, from DIAL (see Appendix 2 for details). Relevant help may be available from your local authority information service. Some past or present experiences may provoke you into joining one of the many local groups campaigning for better local access to public buildings and places.

If you like visiting stately homes and gardens, the *National Trust Handbook* (see Appendix 2) gives information about the suitability of its properties for people in wheelchairs, and there is a separate guide from them for properties that are particularly suitable. All give free admission to someone escorting a person in a wheelchair, and some have motorized buggies for those with mobility problems.

Three other books give details of wheelchair access:

- *Places that care* by Michael Yarrow
- *The National Gardens Scheme handbook*, and
- *Historic houses, castles and gardens*

which list over 1300 properties of all types and gives information about access. Other possible sources of information are RADAR (the Royal Association for Disability and Rehabilitation), and local disability groups, or your local MS Society may have information about access issues to places near to you.

Holidays

If you plan your holiday carefully, you should have no major problems with travelling. Try and stick to a schedule that is not too demanding and, perhaps just as important, allow yourself time to rest at the other end. You might also consult your doctor when you are planning your journey to see if he or she has helpful advice. By and large most airlines are very good at providing extra help and assistance for people with disabilities, including those in wheelchairs, as long as they are notified well in advance of your requirements.

There are a range of tips and advice for longer journeys and holiday travel. If you have vision problems and you are travelling by car, you could enlarge any maps or written instructions before your journey begins. You could also use a highlighter pen on the map to mark out your journey or a magnifying glass with a light on to help you see the map.

In relation to air travel make sure that you give notice on any special requirements you have (such as meals) well in advance. Many airports have motorized 'buggies' to transport people with disabilities. Do take advantage of these, and of porters if you can – you do not want to be too tired out before you have even got on the plane! Ask at the check-in (but preferably before) to try and ensure that your seat allows you to get in and out, and to move as freely as you can. If you take your wheel-chair or scooter with you, do make sure that it is properly and securely labelled and, if it has to be disassembled for travel, it might be wise to take the assembly instructions with you in case someone else has to assemble it again.

If you are travelling overseas take a copy of your passport and any other key documents with you. You might find it helpful, if you are travelling with a companion, to have a change of clothes in each other's luggage, just in case one of the bags is lost – it has happened! Take a special pillow with you for comfort on an aircraft or elsewhere. You might also want to take a small free-standing mirror with you. If you are in a wheelchair, most mirrors are often hard to get close to. Also a soap on a rope is useful.

Investigate whether laundry facilities are available at your place of stay – if they are, you can often take fewer clothes with you. Obviously do check in advance whether your hotel, guest house or motel has any specially prepared rooms for people with disabilities, and especially people in wheelchairs.

There are now a strikingly wide range of support services and organizations for people with MS, almost whatever their disabilities, who wish to take holidays at home or abroad. The key, as we have noted is to plan well in advance, and undertake thorough research about where, and particularly how, you wish to go.

Information on holidays for those with any form of disability can be obtained from a number of sources and there are a rapidly increasing number of sites on the internet giving wide-ranging information (see Appendix 1 for some good websites). Perhaps a feature of these and other sites is what many people might think of as increasingly adventurous holidays for people with disabilities from skiing to sailing. For sailing the Jubilee Sailing Trust has for many years been offering active sailing holidays for those with disabilities as well as able-bodied people on its two tall ships; it also has a very comprehensive list of the websites of other disability organizations.

There are an increasing number of specialist services who can help people with disabilities including, for example, Assistance Travel and Accessible Travel. Other services are increasingly being set up to assist people, not just with MS, who may require special assistance or support in arranging their holidays.

Taking medicines abroad

You should check that you have an appropriate supply of any drugs you are taking whilst you are abroad, for it may not be easy to obtain additional supplies. Sometimes it can be difficult to find a doctor with the necessary expertise, and drug availability and drug licensing conditions are often different. Some drugs may not be readily available – even on prescription in some countries – and certain drugs may only be prescribable by particular kinds of doctor (hospital specialists, for example). Some medicines really need to be kept cool so you may need a 'cool bag' to ensure that they are not spoilt.

It may help to have a letter from your doctor explaining what drugs you are on and what they are for, to avoid possible customs problems, or if you need further supplies in the country to which you are travelling. Customs may well be very interested in your supply of needles if you self-inject, so a letter could get you out of trouble! If you feel you are a bit forgetful, or even if you are not, it is a good idea to divide your supplies into two, placing them in separate bags or suitcases just in case yours gets lost or mislaid. If you wear glasses, take your optician's prescription with you in case you lose them. For general information, the Department of Health produces a leaflet called the *Traveller's Guide to Health* (see Appendix 2). It is also worth repeating that you should have adequate health insurance, and be sure to list MS among what insurance companies call 'pre-existing medical conditions'.

Financial help

There are some organizations that you can apply to if you need financial help for a holiday, although it is important to say that help will be based on your circumstances. These include:

- the Holiday Care Service
- the MS Society, both locally and nationally (although funds are limited)
- some local authorities, and
- local charities.

Your local library or Citizens' Advice should be a good source of information. They may have *The Charities Digest* and *A Guide to Grants for Individuals in Need* and other useful reference books. See Appendices 1 and 2 for details and addresses.

17
Pregnancy, childbirth and the menopause

Issues concerning pregnancy and childbirth often worry people with MS and their partners, as many will have recently embarked on relationships in which they will be considering the possibility of having children. Bringing up children is also another area that concerns both people with MS and those close to them. We also discuss problems older women might encounter.

Pregnancy

Do discuss both your plans and any worries that you have with doctors, and other professional staff looking after you. Pregnancy and childbirth is a time for continuing support. You can receive good advice, and possibly information about sympathetic obstetricians, from the local branch of the MS Society or other MS support groups.

In the past there was often very clear and very negative advice given about pregnancy to someone with MS. In general now this view has changed. A useful way to proceed is to discuss with your partner and/or family and close friends, a series of 'What if?' questions, considering, for example, some of the problems that might occur financially or in relation to child care. Through these means you can rehearse some of the ways of managing potential difficulties, in the hope, and in many cases the expectation, that such problems will not occur.

Relapses tend to be lower in number during pregnancy, and overall most women find their pregnancy is relatively uneventful from an MS point of view.

Feeling good

Many women with MS feel really well while pregnant and would like that feeling to continue afterwards! What is almost certainly happening is that some immunosuppression is occurring naturally in your pregnancy, and lowering the levels of MS activity. So far it has not been possible to identify any of the specific hormones or proteins produced in pregnancy that produce this effect, although one pregnancy hormone has been identified, which suppresses an experimental form of MS in the guinea pig. So there is some basis for optimism in this line of research. However, applying animal-based research to humans has been a notoriously fickle and unpredictable process, so it would be unwise to expect immediate developments as far as people with MS are concerned. On the other hand there is an increased risk of relapse of your MS after delivery and if you should suffer a miscarriage (see below).

Taking drugs

As an important general rule you should not take any drug, even an over-the-counter drug, during pregnancy, or indeed when you are considering becoming pregnant, without discussing this first with your doctor. For many drugs used to treat the everyday symptoms of MS, there is substantial information available about the consequences of their use during pregnancy, and many of them are safe to use.

Those drugs that are now being used to treat the disease itself, rather than any one specific symptom, such as the interferon-based drugs (such as Avonex, Betaferon and Rebif) and Copaxone, are powerful immuno-suppressants, and it is still not clear what effects they will have on an unborn baby. You should stop taking such drugs once you have started trying for a baby, for it will be some time before you know you are pregnant and in the meantime the fertilized egg could be developing. It is a question of balancing your own concerns about the effects of MS on you, and the health of your unborn baby. The decision may not be an easy one to make, but most mothers treat the health of their unborn baby as their main concern at this time.

Childbirth

Miscarriage and relapse

Women with MS run an increased risk of a relapse after a miscarriage as well as after delivery of a baby at the expected time. Miscarriage occurs quite commonly (about a third of all pregnancies miscarry), although many of these miscarriages occur so early in pregnancy that you may not realize what has happened. There is, however, no evidence that a larger number of pregnancies – or a large number of miscarriages – result in any worse outcome as far as MS is concerned.

Delivery problems

Some women with MS who have muscular weakness in their legs or lower bodies, or who may have spasms, might need some assistance with childbirth – perhaps an epidural anaesthesia, for example, or the use of forceps or even a caesarean. However, there is little evidence that MS causes major additional changes in the way that babies are delivered compared to those of women without MS.

The general experience in relation to women with MS is that their pattern of delivery is no different from that of other women. The overall advice for women with MS in relation to preparing for the birth is the same for all women. Prenatal classes, run by your local midwives, and often also by the National Childbirth Trust, would be useful both for you and your partner if you have one, so that you can be taken through the stages of labour and how best to manage them. It may also be worth discussing techniques of pain relief with your midwife and the obstetrician.

There is one other point that you may need to know. If you have been taking steroids over the past few months, such as Prednisone (generic name prednisolone) – and this is one of the drugs that pregnant women have taken safely – then it is possible during the delivery that you will need an extra dose of this drug. This is because during labour the adrenal gland may be 'overloaded', if you have taken steroid drugs over the preceding months, and an additional dose, a 'boost', is needed. This issue ought to be raised with your midwife, and with the obstetrician before the delivery itself, so that they are aware of the situation.

Breastfeeding

If you decide not to breastfeed your baby, you can start taking your drugs again shortly after the delivery of the baby. If you decide to breastfeed, then you do need to seek your doctor's advice – for drugs may be passed to the baby in breast milk.

Breastfeeding is generally recognized as giving the baby the best possible food in the first few months. Of course breastfeeding is only a part of an often exhausting experience that all women have in caring for a newborn baby. If you can, arrange for someone else to help you in the first few weeks after the birth, and whilst it is important – if you wish to continue breastfeeding – to undertake all the feeding yourself in the first 2 or 3 weeks, someone else could help with the particularly exhausting night-time feeds with previously expressed breast milk, or with a relevant formula feed.

Just to reiterate, it is important to be very careful about drugs you are taking during breastfeeding, for they may be passed to the baby through breast milk. With the newer interferon-based drugs and copolymer (Copaxone), you must seek your doctor's advice and you may have to consider not breastfeeding your baby, if you take these drugs.

Other women's issues and the menopause

Urinary symptoms

One of the problems that women with MS face is that they might put almost any symptom they have down to the MS, and concern themselves less about other possibilities. As a general rule, it is important to have any significant symptom you have medically examined. Of particular importance to women is that any urinary symptoms are fully examined, for there is growing evidence that, although many such symptoms are neurological in origin, and are difficult to treat directly, many others are the result of urinary infections, which are, for the most part, treatable. Indeed, if left untreated, such infections can lead to other significant problems.

Routine tests

It is important for women with MS not to neglect other routine tests such as cervical smears and mammograms. If you are taking any immuno-suppressive drugs, such as steroids or interferon-based drugs, you should have such tests more regularly. In a suppressed immune system, it is more likely that precancerous changes will occur in the cervix, for example, and early detection is important.

HRT and the menopause

There doesn't appear to be any evidence that menopausal changes make MS worse, but do discuss the possibilities of hormone replacement therapy (HRT) with your doctor.

The most obvious benefit of HRT is in reducing the possibility of osteoporosis (thinning of the bones) in someone with MS, who may already have mobility problems, and be in danger of falling from time to time. A combination of osteoporosis and increased likelihood of falling might result in fractures that will be difficult to manage. Whether you have HRT or not, you should have a good intake of calcium, both before and after the menopause. A daily intake of at least 1000 mg is recommended before the menopause, and 1500 mg after it. Dairy products are the easiest way to increase calcium intake, although you may obtain calcium from a range of other calcium-fortified products, or calcium supplements.

Other possible benefits of HRT may include:

- decreased vaginal dryness;
- reduced risk for colon cancer and Alzheimer's disease;
- possible reduced risk of heart disease;
- possible benefits in certain forms of incontinence.

Disadvantages of HRT may include the continuation of periods, although usually these are light, and there is still some uncertainty about whether HRT increases the risk of breast cancer, although recent research has suggested that a slightly elevated risk occurs only after several years of use of HRT, and that the first 4 or 5 years of use are not associated with an elevated risk. In addition you may feel that HRT is yet another drug you are taking on top of others to manage various aspects of your MS.

18
Research

Research on the causes, possible cures and ways of managing MS has increased dramatically in recent years. Much of the information that has advanced our understanding of MS has come from what is called basic research – general knowledge of how the brain and central nervous system work and, more recently, how susceptibility to disease may be transmitted genetically. By research, we mean scientific research predominantly conducted by universities, scientific research centres and pharmaceutical (drug) companies. Results of this work are normally published in scientific journals through a process called 'peer review', which means that the work is always subject to critical scrutiny and assessment by other scientists. Through this means, new ideas or theories about MS can be thoroughly evaluated and tested.

Types of research

People sometimes use the term 'research' in a very loose way for almost any kind of information-gathering about a topic of interest – finding out information about your MS, by reading this book for example. However, 'scientific research' involves a very particular way of acquiring information, where a specific question – called a hypothesis – is devised and tested, to find out whether, under particular conditions, that question is answered negatively or positively. To be treated as scientifically correct (valid), the same answer must be repeated under exactly the same conditions by other researchers.

There are broadly five kinds of scientific research being undertaken in relation to MS:

- The systematic study of the distribution and patterns of MS in different communities and countries – usually known as **epidemiological research** – might involve asking questions about whether MS is more common in one geographical area than another, or is decreasing or increasing in a particular population over time, and what factors might explain these differences.

- **Laboratory-based research** focuses on questions related to the development of MS, for example why and how it affects specific nervous system tissue, where researchers often work at the level of individual cells; or what are the possible genetic differences between people with and without MS where blood or tissue types are examined.
- **Clinical research** on patients seeks to answer questions about what is often called the 'natural development' of MS in individuals, through the investigation of particular symptoms and signs that develop in those individuals over time, and what consequences these have for people's ability to function in everyday life.
- Other research concentrates on questions about the effectiveness of potential therapies for MS, commonly undertaken through **clinical trials** – often after extensive safety testing in the laboratory. People with MS may be asked if they wish to participate in a clinical trial, for example to test a new drug.
- More research is increasingly taking place in what is called **applied science** in relation to MS. In the absence of a cure, much of this research is investigating how, for example, physiotherapy or speech therapy can reduce the impact of symptoms, or how far psychological support or counselling can help people to manage their symptoms better.

Each of these approaches uses scientific methods to understand MS, and assist people with the disease. However, the most common form of scientific method you are likely to come across personally is the clinical trial.

Epidemiological research

As we have said, epidemiological research primarily focuses on the distribution of MS in specific populations and countries. In Chapter 1 we talked about some distribution patterns that had led to important lines of inquiry about possible causes of the disease. Thus the facts that MS is found largely in temperate regions of the world and more amongst women, and that there appear to be geographical 'hotspots' of the disease, all seem to explain something about MS. The problem with epidemiological research is that there are many, many reasons why such patterns could occur. Most patterns are misleading in that they either disappear when subjected to detailed investigation, or are explained by another factor not related to MS. Quite a number of people with MS have found several others with the condition in their area, or have had some job or other life experience in common. It is tempting to jump immediately to the conclusion that there must be some link that has caused the MS. Usually such patterns occur just by chance – even when very odd things happen, such as two or three unrelated people with MS living in the same street. In such cases the findings of epidemiological research are primarily suggestive, and must be supported by other kinds of research.

At present two of the most interesting, although very time-consuming, types of epidemiological research, are those trying to detect and assess all people with MS in a particular area, and those measuring the distribution in the population of certain genetic 'markers' linked with MS. In the former studies, findings are indicating that there are more people with MS than we had previously thought, and the latter findings are suggesting increasingly firm associations between particular genetic markers and types of MS.

Laboratory research

There is a very wide spectrum of research in this area; it is usually undertaken on individual cells or cellular processes, often in animals. Much of this research is linked to understanding how the body's immune system in MS seems to attack itself. Many scientists believe that the body's failure to distinguish between 'foreign invaders' in the form of bacteria, viruses and so on (which it should attack), and its own tissue (which it should not attack), is the root explanation of why MS occurs. This kind of research has identified many of the different types of cell in the immune system, how they work, and what happens when they fail or become disrupted. Studying how immune systems work both in animals and in people with MS, who also have other diseases thought to be immune related (such as rheumatoid arthritis), gives a clearer idea of what is happening in people with MS. However, such work is not always directly transferable to MS. For example, in the late 1980s, research on a disease model in animals (called EAE – experimental allergic encephalomyelitis), thought to be similar to MS in humans, revealed promising clues to therapies that might prevent EAE in animals, and thus possibly prevent MS in humans. However, it turned out that the human immune system was far more complicated than that of laboratory animals. As a parallel development a number of fierce immunosuppressant therapies were devised, in the hope that, by suppression of the activities of the immune system, then at least no further 'autoimmune' attacks would occur on the body's own tissue. However, many of these therapies suppressed all immune system activity, and so led to major infections and complications, in which often the intended 'cures' produced worse symptoms than those of the disease they were supposed to help.

Nevertheless, from these studies have come some interesting developments – and one of these developments is work on what are called 'cytokines'. These are chemical messengers associated with the regulation of immune system activity; understanding these cytokines has already proved rewarding. For example 'interferons' are one kind of cytokine and, of course, 'beta-interferons' have proved to give considerable therapeutic benefit in MS. However, the position is still complicated, for some cytokines seem to make MS worse and some seem to help control it; whilst beta-interferons seem to help MS, other types of interferon do not. The lesson from this particular kind of research, just as in much scientific research, is that there are many disappointments as well as new developments, and often the disappointments lead to new approaches to MS.

Clinical research

Clinical research directly involves studying people with MS and their symptoms on an individual basis. Although it may sound strange after many years of research on MS, what is called the 'natural history' of the disease is still not entirely clear, although major studies in Canada have revealed much about the long-term outcome of MS. As we discussed in Chapter 1, it is still not really possible to give anyone a clear idea of how their disease will develop over time, so much clinical research is still devoted to assessing people with MS over long periods of time – several decades – to chart as carefully as possible how their disease develops, especially in relation to early symptoms and signs. Such information is very important, in order to judge, for example, whether early intervention will affect the later course of the disease. As people with the condition know, the effects of MS appear to be very fickle on a day-to-day basis, let alone a longer term one, so it is one of the most difficult research tasks to determine the specific effects of MS, as against those occurring from other, perhaps unrelated, conditions, and the effects of natural ageing processes. Other clinical research is focused on improving and developing diagnostic techniques to try and ensure that such techniques are both accurate and available as early as possible.

Applied research

The traditional kind of research on MS has focused on the causes and cures of the disease, and indeed this kind of research is still the most important in terms of size and funding. However, this research generally does not tackle all the everyday problems that people with MS have of living with the condition. To put it another way, whilst waiting for a cure, people with MS have had to live for years with many difficult and annoying problems, and indeed may have to wait many more years before MS and its problems are banished. Thus an area of 'applied research' has arisen where the focus is on researching the best ways in which people with MS can live with or manage their current and future symptoms, and their consequences. This research might include:

- clinical trial research on drugs and other means of managing everyday symptoms;
- the most appropriate forms of equipment that people may need, to live as comfortably as possible;
- the most effective ways in which physiotherapy, occupational therapy and speech therapy can help people with MS;
- the most appropriate ways in which issues of employment, housing and insurance can be dealt with;
- the psychological and social consequences of MS, especially in relation to concerns about the quality of life, and
- issues about counselling and support for the family consequences of the condition.

In practice, this broad area of 'applied research' is one of the most significant of current research areas, and is one which – on reflection – many people with MS find extremely valuable and relevant. Although everyone wishes to find a cure for MS, a realistic view is that this will take some time, and meanwhile research on how people with MS can make the best of their everyday lives is very important.

Clinical trials

Much of the hugely expensive development work on new (drug) therapies is undertaken by pharmaceutical companies. The commercial return on their investment in these costs, including clinical trials, has to come from patenting and protecting the rights to the therapy involved. Potential medicines that may be freely available, or are not patentable, offer very little incentive for such companies to invest in them, unless they can in some way lay claim to a variant of the medicine concerned or a particular way of administering it. In such cases, other funding agencies, such as the Medical Research Council (MRC), step in to support formal trials on drugs or other substances that are considered promising therapies for MS.

What is a clinical trial?

A clinical trial is actually a formal scientific means of testing the safety or the effectiveness of a drug or other treatment, either against another drug or treatment, or against what is called a 'placebo', i.e. an inactive substance that cannot be distinguished from the 'real' or active drug by people who are taking part in a trial nor the doctors who are administering it. This way the drug can be tested for efficacy compared to the other drug or substance.

In a clinical trial of a potential therapy for MS, usually one group of patients (the experimental group) receives the active drug or the drug being tested, and another group (the control group) receives the drug against which it is to be compared, or the placebo, the inactive substance.

The two groups of patients should be as similar as possible at the outset of the trial, so that the drug alone will make the difference between the groups. Various characteristics of the two groups of people will be measured before, during and after the trial – typically these will include measures of disability, the number of MS 'attacks' or 'relapses' people have had, and other things such as blood cell counts or hormone levels. It is always hoped, of course, that the trial will show that the group who has received the active drug will do better. Thus, for the active drug to be shown to be effective, the trial must finally result in a statistically significant difference between the characteristics of the two groups. However, many trials are relatively inconclusive and, because MS is a complicated condition, statistically significant differences will be observed for some characteristics but not others, or indeed only for certain types of participant.

Blinded and randomised clinical trials

'Blinded' in this sense means that you do not know which drug – active or inactive – you are taking, and thus you will not be able to exert any psychological impact on the results, or be tempted to take supplements if you know that you are in the control rather than the experimental group. People are also usually 'randomized', meaning that they are allocated to either the experimental or control groups randomly, i.e. they cannot choose which group they join. If people are allowed to choose which group they go into, biases may arise in the trial, as certain people, for example with milder or more serious forms of MS, may elect to join one of the groups and not the other. 'Double-blinded' means that the researchers also do not know which people receive which substance. The placebo and the active substance must therefore look and taste identical, so they are often provided in coded containers to each person. Only at the end of the trial is the code broken to reveal who received which compound, when the trial is 'unblinded'. This minimizes the possibility of researchers influencing the outcome, for instance by paying more attention, or giving additional and differential care, to people in the treatment group during the trial.

The placebo effect

The 'placebo effect', i.e. feeling better as a result of taking any 'medication' that people believe may have a beneficial effect whatever its real and unique (physiological) effects, has been shown to operate even when coloured water is drunk. Therefore there is a danger that any real effects of a drug being tested could be mixed up with this 'placebo effect', which is why *comparing* treatments in identical ways is so important. Indeed, the problem caused by the placebo effect is one reason why rigorous clinical trials must be performed before a new drug or other therapy can be scientifically accepted.

Clinical trial phases

Before a drug can be licensed for normal clinical use, there are three essential sets of information that have to be researched: its safety (a Phase 1 trial), its appropriate dose levels and the medical conditions or symptoms for which it is best suited (a Phase II trial), and its effectiveness (a Phase III trial).

- A **Phase I clinical trial** is a test of safety, or toxicity, and is aimed primarily at determining whether the substance has any adverse effects on humans. Of course, before the drug is given to humans, toxicity will also have been tested in animals, cell cultures or computer simulation tests.
- A **Phase II clinical trial** is usually only undertaken on a small scale and determines whether a larger scale trial is worth undertaking. Phase II trials also help to clarify which groups of people and, for example, which types of MS are most likely to benefit, and how that benefit might be measured. However, Phase II trials may not test for effectiveness, which often requires large numbers of subjects.
- So a **Phase III trial** is necessary to prove the effectiveness of a drug to enable it to be licensed for clinical practice. Phase III trials are

usually very large, very expensive and very lengthy, but show to a high degree of statistical certainty how effective a substance is in treating the chosen people and conditions.

- Sometimes **Phase IV trials** are undertaken. These are conducted after the drug has been licensed, and thus may be described as the 'post-marketing phase' of trials. In such trials, longer term side effects may be assessed; the drug may be tested in different types of MS; or its use may be tested in other conditions – perhaps not associated with MS.

Of course it is important to say that, even when a drug has been tested in all three Phases (I,II and III) and is licensed for clinical use, it may still not become widely available owing to its cost, practical problems in administering it, or its generally unacceptable side effects.

Which drugs are tested in clinical trials?

As we have implied, in order for a drug to be licensed for clinical use, it has to go through the complicated process of clinical trials, and such a process is very expensive. Increasingly, international pharmaceutical companies sponsor the majority of such trials, with additional support from national Multiple Sclerosis Societies, and government-funded Medical Research Councils. Whilst pharmaceutical companies necessarily use scientific methods to evaluate the drugs that they themselves have developed, the choices as to which are subjected to the most expensive Phase III trials, or indeed the initial choices as to which drugs are developed, must – in their terms – be subject to a commercial judgement on their part. This would involve making a judgement about the size of the market for such a drug, and its likely profitability, as well as, of course, making a judgement about its likely efficacy.

It would be reassuring to believe that only a scientific basis was used to decide which drugs were subject to Phase III trials, but generally there are far more drugs that could be subject to such trials than the funding available, and it is clear that commercial as well as scientific factors must intrude in the selection process. Such a process, at least from a commercial point of view, is likely to relegate drugs with a potentially low profitability, or which cannot be patented. The history of therapeutic possibilities in MS is littered with the hopes of people often for non-patentable substances in relation to the disease – such as evening primrose oil, hyperbaric oxygen and, most recently, cannabis. It is very unlikely that pharmaceutical companies would be involved in testing such substances unless they can patent a variant of the substance concerned, and thus usually – as in the case of all three substances mentioned – medical charities and/or the government-funded Medical Research Councils themselves would need to fund such trials. Such funding may occur in response to the continuous and widely expressed concerns of people with MS, although decisions for this kind of funding are not normally justified on this basis.

Finally, it is worth saying that, although some major potential therapeutic advances will remain untested because of the particular focus of the pharmaceutical companies, this is unlikely because of the significant number of checks and balances made by the Multiple Sclerosis Society and the Medical Research Council.

Participating in a clinical trial

First of all it is important to say that, if you participate in a clinical trial (especially a Phase III trial) for MS, it will generally not be guaranteed that you will receive the new drug – but you will indeed have *a chance* to take it, probably on the basis of being randomized to the 'treatment group'. You will probably have a 50–50 chance of receiving the new drug or being randomized into the 'control' group, who will use either a placebo or another comparison drug.

However, there are several reasons why it is still worth your while joining a clinical trial, even if you are not given the new drug by being randomized to a comparison group:

- To be frank, it is likely that you will receive more careful clinical assessment and support, than you otherwise would do, if you participate in a clinical trial, *whether you receive the new drug or not*. This is because all those participating have to be meticulously and regularly monitored.
- You will almost certainly gain from the placebo effect, whatever you are taking in the trial.
- You would have the altruistic satisfaction of participating in a trial that would benefit others, even if you do not have the new drug yourself.
- Often trial procedures allow standard tried and tested therapies to continue to be used if, for example, you have an attack or exacerbation during the trial.
- More frequently now, trials compare one drug with another, not just with a placebo substance. In these trials you would receive an active drug, whichever group you were in. Indeed the comparison drug will already have been shown to effective in managing some aspects of MS, and often the new drug is one in which only a marginal additional assistance for MS is hoped for – but not yet known.

Depending on the type of clinical trial concerned, people are used from many different sources, but the largest sources of all are people with MS already under the care of neurologists, or those who are attending hospital clinics. In Britain the major means of recruitment is usually directly through your neurologist. When they are notified of a particular trial, they will investigate their own lists of people with MS to see whether any are suitable for the trial. You would then be contacted and asked if you would be prepared to participate. Of course, you can make your neurologist aware of your interest in clinical trials at one of your assessment meetings or by letter. Increasingly, in the United States, trials are more widely advertised through specialist centres and publications, and people can apply directly to participate, but in Britain this more open process of recruitment is still in its infancy.

Eligibility

One of the things about clinical trials is that they all have what are called eligibility criteria. These are often very specific, and relate to the particular types of people and the particular types of MS that they feel would most benefit from the new drug. These criteria could mean that your type of MS is not considered to be the type that could gain most from the new drug. There is also another consideration here. In order to be able to test for the effectiveness of a drug over a reasonable period of time, people whose MS is currently changing relatively rapidly, or who are having attacks, or in whom progression is more measurable (for example in relation to changes in the ability to walk) may well be chosen, in preference to people whose MS is worse overall but is relatively stable. Thus it is often frustrating for people with long-standing MS to be excluded from some trials, on the grounds that they cannot walk, or that their MS is too advanced. However, more recently, for such people who wish to participate in clinical trials, some of the newer interferon family of drugs, and indeed others, are now being tested on people with longer term and progressive MS. Do not to get too disheartened if you are not eligible for one clinical trial, because there may be others you can join in due course.

Payment for drugs

You should not be asked to pay for any drugs you receive in clinical trials in which you participate. As a matter of principle, either pharmaceutical companies or other funding bodies of trials pay for these drugs. Indeed your travelling expenses will usually be reimbursed if, for example, you need to attend for assessment at a hospital more frequently for the trial than you would otherwise have done.

There is one issue of payment, however, that sometimes arises, and that is at the conclusion of a trial, when a new drug may be found to be effective, and participants wish to continue taking it. Usually trial funding bodies will not pay for any continuing administration of the drug beyond the end of trial, and you would have to negotiate any such administration through your usual doctor. In many cases this may be difficult, not only because new drugs may be very expensive but also because they may not yet be licensed for clinical use outside a trial.

Patient consent

It is a requirement for participation in all properly conducted trials that you – as a potential participant – give your 'informed consent'. You will have received a form and almost certainly have had a discussion with your doctor, and this form states the nature, benefits and risks of the trial, and asks you formally to give your consent to participation in the trial. You are also agreeing to follow the procedures that the trial requires. The form should be written in clear and plain English, and usually Ethics Committees, who give necessary ethical approval for such trials, try and make sure that such forms are not written in medical or legal jargon. If there is anything, anything at all, that is not clear in the document, then it is essential that you ask for clarification before agreeing to participate.

Some recent trials on beta-interferon

The results of some recent clinical trials have shown that the beta-interferons may slow down the course of the disease over a 3–4-year period. We must remember that the criteria for 'relapsing-remitting MS' in trials are drawn very tightly and many people have types of MS that were not covered by previous trial findings. New trials are underway to test whether these other people might benefit as well. However, because it is more difficult to test the effects of such drugs in people with more complicated relapsing-remitting, or progressive types of MS, the findings are taking some time, although initial results are promising. The difficulty is turning out to be not just the *effectiveness* of interferons in these cases but their *cost effectiveness*. Although it has been shown that interferons may slow down the disease in some people, the number in which this occurs is not large, and the costs of the drugs are very expensive. A number of clinicians and also, importantly, other bodies regulating the extent to which the drugs can be used on the NHS for such types of MS were reluctant to see it made available for all categories. Now there is agreement with the pharmaceutical industry to share expenses of the treatment.

Previous trials on steroids

One trial on steroid therapy has indicated that the steroids reduced the risk of developing clinically definite MS by half over a 2-year period. There have been serious criticisms of some aspects of the trial, and further trials are needed on this issue. However, further trials to test whether this was an abnormal result or not are very difficult to organize. It is almost impossible to identify and ensure that enough people participate in such a trial with very early, and especially the first, symptoms of MS, i.e. within a month or so of those symptoms appearing – and also to ensure that they have an MRI scan within this phase. Because the beta-interferons and other drugs have shown more overall promise in MS, there is now some reluctance to conduct large-scale and expensive trials on steroids.

New lines of research

Genetic research

Chapter 1 discusses the possible causal relationship between MS, genetics and the environment. The most striking thing now is the speed at which research on possible underlying genetic factors is being undertaken. Of course, this research is part of the massive international research effort which has now 'mapped' human genetic makeup – in other words which has unravelled the human 'genome'. In the course of this research more and more genetic associations with particular diseases are being uncovered. Of particular interest is the fact that genes control the human immune system, and so, if it turns out that people with MS have a clearly different genetic makeup to other people, ultimately the most effective way to manage immune system malfunctions may be to try and deal with those genetic differences. This will not be a simple process because several genes are already known to be implicated in MS, unlike some other conditions where only one gene is involved.

Currently genetic research on MS is based on two main lines of inquiry:

- Genes that allow the body to recognize which are its own tissues and which are those of an 'invader' bacteria or virus are being studied. If this recognition process goes wrong, then an 'autoimmune' attack of the body's own tissue is likely to occur, as in MS. The genes under investigation here that perform this recognition function – 'histocompatibility genes' – are usually either HLA (human leukocyte antigen) genes, or MHC (major histocompatibility) genes.

- The genetic control of 'lymphocytes' (T cells), which are one important class of cells responding to insults to the immune system, is the second line of study. Although there is much detailed research still to be undertaken, it appears likely that a combination of genes controlling these lymphocytes and related immune activity produces a susceptibility in people with MS to the disease, although other triggering factors, perhaps environmentally determined, may be necessary for the onset of the disease.

Research on viruses and MS

The relationship of viruses to MS has been the subject of much research over the past two decades, and causes an equal amount of controversy. Almost every year, it has been claimed that a virus specific to the cause of MS has been discovered. However, none of these claims has been sustained after further extensive investigation. The basic issue is really one of cause or effect. Does a virus cause MS, or does a weakened immune system have the effect of making the body more susceptible to attack by viruses? Most researchers believe the latter to be the case, but an existing faulty recognition process in the immune system may either also fail to recognize (and thus attack) an invading virus, or such a virus may, through the same process, accelerate the body's own attack on itself. In this respect recent work on viruses is being linked to other research on malfunctioning immune systems, and genetic research is also continuing.

Regeneration of myelin

This research area – trying to regenerate myelin – has been significant over the past few years. The cells that produce myelin are called 'oligodendrocytes', one of a family of what are described as 'glial cells'. If the life of oligodendrocytes could be fully understood, as well as their role in the formation and repair of myelin, then an attempt to encourage their revitalization in MS could be made. This research process has also involved investigating exactly how the nervous system responds to myelin damage and how scar tissue is formed, as well as estimating what effects regeneration of myelin might have.

Research on myelin damage and possible regeneration is yet another story of an initially hopeful scientific development followed by major disappointment. For some time it was thought that myelin could not be regenerated at all, and then more sophisticated techniques indicated that myelin repair did occur in MS, although it was very slow and weak – and was not enough to compensate for the original damage. Now scientists are concentrating on seeing whether and how this process of repair might be made more effective. The importance of this research is the knowledge that, even if myelin has been lost (and thus messages along the nerves are malfunctioning), the underlying nervous tissue is almost certainly still intact, at least in the early stages of MS; thus, if it was reinsulated (remyelinated), it may well be able to function normally. Once demyelination has occurred for some time this may be less likely.

Animal models have suggested that remyelination is possible in such a way as to restore some functions originally lost. Strategies have included:

- using substances called *growth factors* to enhance the actions of myelin-producing cells;
- trying to inhibit other processes that weaken the actions of those cells, or
- in a more adventurous way, investigating the possibility of transplanting cells to produce myelin.

There are a number of substances being tested on humans to assist remyelination, although the lessons of the disappointments of equally promising possibilities arising from animal work with EAE (see above) are important to bear in mind. It is also important to say that most of the remyelinating strategies are essentially compensatory ones, i.e. they do not address the underlying disease process that is still going on – whilst some remyelination may be assisted, other demyelination may be occurring or about to occur. In addition for those with long-standing MS, the underlying nervous tissue will probably have been damaged, as well as the myelin coating of that tissue. In such a situation, remyelination may have little or no effect on symptoms.

Finding out more

There is a variety of sources about new research on MS. Which you use depends on your own inclinations, and indeed your own resources! The most important source of reliable and accurate scientific research on MS is that contained in the peer-reviewed scientific, and especially neurological, journals. Usually these are not obtainable directly except in specialist medical libraries, but recent key issues and findings on MS from the journals can be obtained through computer searches, often through ordinary libraries, using one of the major medical databases such as

'Medline'. Increasingly the MS Society in Britain, and the MS Society in the United States are putting out press statements and information on major current research issues, often highlighting advances in their regular Newsletters.

If you have access to the World Wide Web, there are now all sorts of possibilities of keeping track of new research. These include:

- the websites of the MS Society in Britain and the United States;
- the website of MS Trust, which is fast, efficient and up to date;
- using one of the 'search engines' on the Web to trawl for updates on MS, and other sources of information;
- joining ones of the growing number of Newsgroups in which people exchange information about new developments and other issues about MS. These latter groups are particularly important in terms of contact with other people with MS, and are often likely to be amongst the first sources of information about all kinds of developments, both scientific and non-scientific.

Web addresses are currently changing too fast to permit any sensible listing here, but one source which is likely to be with us for sometime is the Usenet News Group at news://alt.support.mult-sclerosis. This group hosts 50–100 messages per day and includes announcements about new web pages and updates about existing pages.

The next stage beyond these publications is to go to a good public library (a regional centre rather than a local library) and search for books on MS. Most libraries, including most local public libraries now have computer terminals for keyword and title searches. Library staff are usually keen to help with difficult searches and to help locate specific information.

Glossary

ACTH (adrenocorticosteroid hormone) This hormone reduces inflammation. Clinical trials in the 1970s and later showed that it reduced the length of relapses or exacerbations in MS. More recently, a different family of steroids (glucocorticosteroids) has been found to have fewer side effects, as well as generally being more effective. So ACTH is used less in MS than previously, although some neurologists feel that ACTH still has significant value in treating MS relapses.

action tremor An involuntary trembling or shaking of a muscle or muscle group which is more noticeable during movement than when the muscle is at rest – for instance when reaching for an object or taking a step. Some degree of tremor is normal for all people, but a tremor that interferes with ordinary activity may be a symptom of neuromuscular disorder.

activities of daily living (or ADLs) A set of activities essential to independent living, such as washing, dressing and eating. Some particular sets of activities, as well as formalized procedures for measuring the performance of those activities, have become established as assessments of the degree of disability caused by MS. Such ADL scores may be used to record the progress of MS, to assess domestic needs or to test the effects of drugs in clinical trials.

ambulant Able to walk unassisted, with or without a walking aid (a stick or frame, for instance).

anticholinergic drugs Such drugs are used in the management of urinary problems owing to neurological impairment. The name refers to the way in which the drugs work by affecting the parasympathetic nervous system, reducing spasms (contractions) in the bladder and thus reducing the likelihood of involuntary or too frequent urination.

artefact effect A coincidental association (or one with no cause) between two factors, often explained by a third factor.

atrophy Wasting away or reduction in the size of tissue, particularly muscle tissue, following prolonged disuse.

auditory evoked response An electrical signal in the brain that occurs in response to sound. Tests can reveal changes in the speed, shape and distribution of these signals which are indicative of a diagnosis of MS.

autoimmune disease A disorder of the immune system in which the processes that usually defend against disease run amok and attack the body's own tissues (myelin, in the case of MS). Other autoimmune conditions include rheumatoid arthritis and lupus erythematosus. The systematic study of autoimmune diseases as a group is an important part of research into MS.

benign MS An instance of MS which is either mild (possibly displaying no active symptoms) or in which there is little or no evidence of progressively more severe symptoms.

beta-blockers A class of drugs (known more fully as beta-adrenergic blocking agents) commonly used to treat high blood pressure, irregular heart beat, migraine and angina.

bipolar disorder Also often known as manic-depressive disorder, an illness which is characterized by extreme and unpredictable mood swings.

blood–brain barrier (BBB) A barrier separating the brain from the blood supplying it. In normal circumstances, essential nutrients can cross the barrier from the blood into the brain and waste products cross from the brain into the blood, but the cells of the brain are shielded from potentially harmful substances.

Borrelia burgdorferii The Latin name for the infectious organism that causes Lyme disease, an entirely treatable infection spread by ticks, which has many symptoms in common with MS and can be mistaken for it.

bowel incontinence *see* **faecal incontinence**

bowel regimen A programme involving changes in diet and timing of bowel movements designed to control faecal incontinence. Dietary changes include an increase in fibre and fluid intake to increase the bulk and to soften bowel movements and a reduction in intestinal irritants such as coffee and alcohol. A bowel regimen may also employ laxatives and drugs to help complete emptying of the bowel at predictable times.

Candida albicans Also known as thrush, this is a fungus that is often present in the genitals, mouth and other moist parts of the body. Symptoms of candidiasis include irritation, itching, abnormal discharges and discomfort on passing water. Candidiasis can be effectively treated with antifungal drugs.

cardiovascular Relating to the heart and blood vessels.

cerebrospinal fluid (CSF) The fluid surrounding the spinal column and nerves supplying stimuli to the brain. The CSF contains proteins and tissue fragments that can aid the diagnosis of neurological disorders and differentiate MS from other conditions (such as a haemorrhage) with similar or overlapping symptoms. A sample of CSF can be taken with a spinal tap (*see* **lumbar puncture**).

chi (qi) In Chinese medicine, the essential life-force or energy flowing in the body, imbalance of which results in the symptoms of disease or illness.

chronic progressive (or primary progressive) MS A type of MS characterized by a pattern of progressively more severe or widespread symptoms over time.

cognitive abilities Ability to perform tasks related to thought processes – for instance problem-solving, recognition, memory and recall. Changes in cognitive ability are often subtle and not apparent without sophisticated testing. Cognitive tests may reveal evidence of changes due to MS.

cognitive issues A set of issues relating to such things as memory, information processing, planning and problem solving, which are of recent but rapidly growing significance to the study of MS.

computerized axial tomography (CAT or CT) scan A form of detailed X-ray imaging involving multiple exposures at different positions and angles throughout the same part of the body. Computerized manipulation of the exposures results in clear images of fine structures such as sclerotic plaques within the brain or spinal column.

contractures Shortening or shrinkage of tissue (such as connective or muscular tissue) which may result from inflammation caused by MS and which can restrict movement of joints. Exercises to maintain the flexibility of joints are particularly important because contractures may be made worse by lack of joint use.

dementia Disorder of behaviour and cognitive function causing memory disorders, changes in personality, deterioration in personal care, impaired reasoning and disorientation.

demyelination The biochemical process of damage to the protective sheath surrounding nerves, damage or loss of which leads to symptoms of MS. The breakdown of myelin leads to poor or weak messages to various parts of the body and may lead, in the case of MS, to the formation of plaques or scarring with hardened (sclerotic) tissue.

diplopia Double vision, resulting (in the case of MS) from impaired control of eye muscles.

electroencephalographic (EEG) recordings The measurement of nerve signals within the brain, using electrodes placed harmlessly on the skin of the scalp.

epidemiology The study of patterns of birth, death and disease within and between human populations. Often epidemiological studies try to find relationships between the frequency of MS and variations in other factors (such as diet or exposure to infections).

essential fatty acids Important substances crucial to nervous system development and health. They cannot be synthesized by the body and must be obtained from the diet – these are the families of linoleic, linolenic and arachidonic acids.

euphoria A strong sense of happiness or wellbeing, usually in response to a pleasurable stimulus. However, euphoria without an obvious cause or stimulus may occur in MS.

faecal (bowel) incontinence The involuntary release of faeces from the bowel, resulting from constipation and partial obstruction of the bowel or from diminished control of the anal sphincter. Treatment of faecal incontinence with a bowel regimen is often completely successful in preventing involuntary bowel movements.

familial component A situation in which more relatives have the same disease than would be expected by chance. This can be due to an inherited susceptibility to the disease (nature) or to the environmental and other exposures that families inevitably share (nurture).

family pedigrees A family tree that details the number of instances of disease amongst all members related to each other by blood. Pedigrees are important in determining the mechanisms of genetic inheritance.

foot drop A disorder in which, instead of the normal 'heel then toe' pattern of walking, the toe touches the ground first, leading often to tripping and falling. The condition results from weakness in the ankle and foot muscles, caused by weakening of nervous system control of these muscles.

frequency The desire or need to empty the bladder often.

functional abilities Ability to perform tasks. A number of objective tests have been developed to assess the extent to which these abilities may be affected by the progression of MS.

gait analysis The study of exactly how people walk, which that can be used to assess the effects of MS and the effectiveness of therapies, such as physio-therapy, in helping people to walk more comfortably.

glucocorticosteroids A family of drugs (including prednisone, prednisolone, methyl-prednisolone) which, whilst produced naturally by the adrenal gland, can be made synthetically. They have immunosuppressive and anti-inflammatory properties. They are replacing ACTH for use in MS exacerbations.

hesitancy An involuntary delay or inability to start urinating.

immunosuppressive drugs Drugs which suppress the body's natural immune responses. They have been widely used in MS because immune responses are considered to be directed against the person's own body in the disease.

improved case ascertainment Sometimes people may have MS but it has not been diagnosed. Improved case ascertainment is the increased ability of the medical services to identify correctly such existing cases which have been previously undetected.

incidence of disease The measure of how often new cases of a disease are diagnosed within a population. When the incidence of a disease is low, incidence will be reported per 100,000 people per year.

incontinence Loss of control of bladder or bowel function. Incontinence may result in occasional accidents or in more serious loss of voluntary control of urination or bowel movements.

inoculations *see* **vaccinations**

inpatient Someone who is admitted to a bed in a hospital ward and remains there for a period of time for treatment, examination or observation.

intramuscularly Injections within or into a muscle as opposed to intravenous (directly into a vein) injections.

labile Volatile or unstable. What is called 'emotional lability', i.e. unpredictable or changeable moods, occurs in some people with MS.

latitude effect An often-repeated observation in MS research that there is a relationship between the incidence of MS and the distance from the equator (or latitude in geography). In other words, the further you go from the equator, the more increases in MS cases there are, but cases lessen towards the polar regions. The nature of the relationship has not been fully unravelled, and there many explanations as to why it should exist.

licensed drugs Medicinal compounds licensed by the Medicines Control Agency for general use within medical practice in respect of particular illnesses – in other words, licensed drugs also have licensed purposes. Not all legally available drugs are licensed, such as new and untested drugs as well as some private treatments, supplements and complementary treatments.

lumbar puncture (spinal tap) A procedure in which a hollow needle is inserted into the spinal canal between two vertebrae in the lower back, in order to withdraw a sample of cerebrospinal fluid for biochemical analysis.

magnetic resonance imaging (MRI) A procedure in which a magnetic field, generated inside a large cylinder in which the person to be examined lies, produces detailed images of fine structures within the body. Unlike X-ray imaging, MRI can image soft tissue such as the brain, spinal cord and blood vessels.

major depressive episode A state in which deep sadness and unhappiness may be accompanied by disturbances or major problems in appetite and sleep patterns, plus feelings of hopelessness, worthlessness and suicidal thoughts.

malignant MS As opposed to benign MS, in which progression to more severe or widespread symptoms is very slow or absent, malignant MS progresses clearly and relentlessly. A diagnosis of malignant MS may be made, based on a particularly severe instance of MS, an uncharacteristically rapid progression or the absence of distinct periods of remission. The boundaries between primary progressive and malignant MS are indistinct and dependent upon clinical judgement.

medical history Literally, the file of notes and records about a patient and his or her medical events. The taking of a medical history (the interview in which a doctor asks how an illness or symptoms started) is a crucial first phase in the diagnosis of any condition. In the case of MS, where diagnosis can be a long, tedious and complex procedure, the collection of an accurate and complete medical history is of particular importance.

meridians Lines of energy running through the body, connecting the different anatomical sites, upon which much traditional Chinese medicine is based.

motor symptoms Symptoms relating to muscular movement and the control of motion. Motor symptoms are those symptoms of MS that result from various components of degeneration of nervous system function resulting from MS plaques.

multiple scleroses Scleroses (or sclerotic plaques) are deposits of hardened tissue which can result from inflammation around nerves in the brain or spinal cord (central nervous system). In MS, a sclerosis can result in abnormal and more permanent damage in many parts of the nervous system. In severe MS, there may be many of these scleroses causing loss of control of muscle function.

myelin An electrical insulator covering nerve fibres which ensures that nerve messages are effectively transmitted to various parts of the body. *See also* **demyelination**

neurological examination An evaluation of the function of the nervous system involving, often, a great number of individual examinations and tests. A neurological assessment is essential to the diagnosis of MS, which will (at least initially) involve the elimination of other, often more serious or immediate, conditions with similar symptoms. These may include the taking of a relevant medical history, examination of reflexes, senses and functional abilities, auditory and visual evoked response tests, MRI scans where it is thought their results would significantly aid the diagnosis. An examination of cognitive function (such as memory and problem solving) is becoming more uncommon. A full neurological assessment may take place over many occasions and be spread over many weeks or months.

neurone (or neuron) A nerve cell.

NICE (National Institute of Clinical Excellence) This independent body has recently been established by the British Government to assess the effectiveness of healthcare interventions in relation to their cost. The intention is that only interventions (including drugs) approved by NICE will be available through the NHS.

nocturia The desire or need to pass urine during the night, often disturbing restful sleep.

nystagmus An involuntary, jerking movement of the eyes resulting (in the case of MS) from damage to the nervous system. Nystagmus can result in severe visual problems that make reading extremely tiring or difficult.

oligoclonal banding The banding is distributed discretely in the spinal fluid of a large proportion (90%) of people with MS, although it is not limited to just those. The banding indicates abnormal levels of antibodies.

optic neuritis Inflammation of the optic nerve behind the eye. Optic neuritis can result in temporary loss vision, as well as pain and tenderness.

outpatient Someone who receives treatment at a hospital but is not admitted to a bed in a ward.

paresis Weakness or partial paralysis of muscles.

population ageing A term for the general trend, in all industrialized nations, towards greater life expectancy. Increased life expectancy leads inevitably to a greater proportion of people at all older ages, a greater dependency ratio (the ratio of employed people to children and retired people), and a greater proportion of the population with long-term medical needs. Population ageing and the resulting increased demand for health services will become an increasingly important political issue over coming decades.

prevalence A measure of the proportion of the population with a given condition, often expressed as so many cases of the condition for each thousand people of the population. This measure allows comparison of the frequency of the condition between populations of different sizes.

primary progressive MS *see* **chronic progressive MS**

prognosis An educated assessment of the likely future course of a medical condition and its effects. No prognosis can ever be more than a good guess based on prior experience, and may include both best and worst case outcomes.

progressive neurological disease A disease of the nervous system that becomes progressively more severe or has more widespread symptoms over time.

qi *see* *chi*

recall bias The tendency of those people, when answering questions about past events, to selectively remember past events and circumstances. For instance, people who have a disease affecting their ability to walk may selectively remember more illnesses or accidents affecting their legs compared to other people who may have had an equal number of illnesses or accidents. Recall bias can be a significant problem when researchers are trying to discover past events which may have caused a disease.

relapsing-remitting MS A type of MS which is characterized by relapses, i.e. a relatively rapid increase in symptoms, followed by remissions in which there is a partial or full recovery from these untreated symptoms. In some cases complete recovery may occur from all symptoms, but in most cases recovery is partial. Relapses may recur every few months or may be as much as years apart.

scotoma A 'gap' or large 'blind spot' in one part of your visual field.

secondary progressive MS A type of MS in which, following initially benign or relapsing-remitting MS, symptoms then begin to progress steadily.

selective recall *see* **recall bias**

sensory symptoms Symptoms which involve a problem with one of the senses – touch, taste, smell, hearing and sight. All senses may be affected in MS, although visual and auditory disturbances are most frequently reported and are most likely to impact on activities of daily living.

sequelae The indirect effects of a condition. For instance, urinary tract infections and bed sores are not caused by MS, but can result from immobility and being bedbound, and are more common amongst people with severe symptoms of MS.

shiatzu A form of massage based on the pressure treatment (acupressure) of points associated with acupuncture treatment.

spasticity Stiffness or tension in muscles that is not caused by excessive exercise, and in MS is usually caused by the continuing effect of poor nervous system control of the relevant muscles.

spinal tap *see* **lumbar puncture**

subcutaneously Under the skin, e.g. a subcutaneous injection is given in the tissues immediately beneath the skin.

tremor An involuntary shaking or trembling of muscles, at rest or (more commonly in MS) during movement.

trigeminal neuralgia This is acute pain associated with disorder of the trigeminal nerve – the nerve supplying the cheek, lips, gums and chin. The pain is usually intense, stabbing, brief and associated with only one side of the face.

urgency The desire or need to pass urine immediately. Urgency is not necessarily associated with a full bladder, but is nevertheless almost impossible to ignore.

Uhtoff's phenomenon A temporary disturbance of vision that may follow vigorous exercise.

vaccination A means of producing immunity in a person by using a preparation to stimulate the formation of antibodies, now used synonymously with the word 'inoculation'.

vertigo A disorientating sensation of unsteadiness. The world often appears to be spinning. It may sometimes be described as a dizzy spell. Vertigo results from a disturbance of the fluid in the inner ear or from a disorder of the nerve carrying signals from the inner ear to the brain. Even a simple but unfamiliar situation (such as sailing) can cause vertigo in a healthy person, leading to nausea or vomiting.

vestibular system The system of balance that operates through fluid-filled canals in the inner ear and the nerve carrying signals from the inner ear to the brain.

voiding Literally, emptying. Voiding is usually applied to bowel motions and passing urine. Incomplete voiding refers to the situation where, after a motion or urination, the bowel or bladder is not emptied completely.

Appendix 1
Useful addresses and websites

National and regional MS societies

**Multiple Sclerosis Society of GB
& N. Ireland**
The MS National Centre
372 Edgware Road
London NW2 6ND
Helpline: 0808 800 8000
Tel: 020 8438 0700
Fax: 020 8438 0701
Website: www.mssociety.org.uk
*Offers general information and support to
people with MS and their families. Has local
branches and funds research.*

**Multiple Sclerosis Society:
N. Ireland Office**
The Resource Centre
34 Annadale Avenue
Belfast BT7 3JJ
Tel: 0289 080 2802
Fax: 0289 080 2803
Website: www.mssocietyni.co.uk
*Offers general information and support via
local groups to people with MS and their
families.*

The Multiple Sclerosis Society, Scotland
Ratho Park
88 Glasgow Road
Ratho Station
Edinburgh EH28 8PP
Helpline: 0808 800 8000
Tel: 0131 335 4050
Fax: 0131 335 4051
Website: www.mssociety.org.uk
*General information and local support groups
for people with MS and their families.*

International MS societies

Multiple Sclerosis Society of Canada
250 Bloor Street East
Suite 1000
Toronto
Ontario M4W 3P9
Tel: 00 1 416 922 6065
Fax: 00 1 416 922 7538
Website: www.mssociety.ca
*Organization offering information and
support to people with MS and their families.*

**Multiple Sclerosis International
Federation**
3rd Floor, Skyline House
200 Union Street
London SE1 0LX
Tel: 020 7620 1911
Fax: 020 7620 1922
Website: www.msif.org
*Links research and development projects of
Multiple Sclerosis societies across the world.*

Multiple Sclerosis Society of Ireland
4th Floor
Dartmouth House
Grand Parade
Dublin 6
Tel: 00353 126 94599
Fax: 00353 126 93746
Website: www.ms-society.ie
*General information, telephone counselling
and local support groups for people with MS
and their families. Funds specialized
community workers. Is member of Multiple
Sclerosis International Federation.*

Other MS-related organizations

British Trust for the Myelin Project
Douglas Cottage
1 Drumbrae Gardens
Edinburgh EH12 8SY
Tel: 0131 339 8424
Fax: 0131 339 8439
Website: www.myelinprobritish.demon.co.uk
The Trust is part of an international network which funds, links and shares research projects throughout the world into the repair of myelin and reduction of disabilities.

MS First
MS Research Unit
Bristol General Hospital
Guinea Street
Bristol BS1 6SY
Tel: 0117 928 6332
Fax: 0117 928 6371
Website: ww.digitalbristol/members/msfirst
Supports Bristol MS Research Unit, an internationally recognized research facility within a premier NHS Trust associated with the University of Bristol.

MS Healing Trust
PO Box 2469
Shirley
Solihull B90 2QZ
Tel: 0121 744 7167
Fax: 0121 733 8982
Trust exists to maximize the healing potential in people with MS. It runs a monthly clinic at Shirley attended by doctors, and an information service. Appointments are essential.

Multiple Sclerosis Resource Centre
7 Pear Tree Business Centre
Pear Tree Road
Stanway
Colchester CO3 0JN
Tel: 01206 505444
Fax: 01206 505449
24-hour counselling line: 0800 783 0517
Website: www.msrc.co.uk
Help and advice lines, magazine for people with MS and their families.

Multiple Sclerosis Trust
Spirella Building
Bridge Road
Letchworth SG6 4ET
Tel: 01462 476700
Fax: 01462 476710
Website: www.mstrust.org.uk
Provides information for people with MS, runs professional education courses and funds research into MS management.

Multiple sclerosis therapy centres

National MS Therapy Centres
Bradbury House
155 Barkers Lane
Bedford MK41 9RX
Helpline: 0800 783 0518
Tel: 01234 325781
Fax: 01234 365242
24-hour counselling line: 0800 783 0518
Website: www.ms-selfhelp.org
Umbrella headquarters acting for therapy centres around the UK. Provides various therapies for the management of MS.

Other useful addresses

Able to Go
www.abletogo.com
Offers listings of places to go and rates those places for access and a number of other criteria for disabled travellers.

Abilitynet
PO Box 94
Warwick CV34 5WS
Help Line: 0800 269545
Tel: 01926 312847
Fax: 01926 407425
Website: www.abilitynet.org.uk
Advice and support given to help make the benefits of using computers available to disabled children and adults. Can arrange assessment at home or in the work place for a fee.

Accessible Travel
Avionics House
Naas Lane
Gloucester GL2 2SN
Tel: 01452 729 739
Specializes in supporting people on holidays throughout the UK and the world who need nursing or a range of other support services.

Action for Leisure
c/o Warwickshire College
Moreton Morrell
Warwick CV35 9BL
Tel: 01926 650195
Website: www.actionforleisure.org.uk
Offers information about activities, equipment and local opportunities. Promotes play and leisure for people with disabilities of all ages.

Age Concern England
Astral House
1268 London Road
London SW16 4ER
Help Line: 0800 009966
Tel: 020 8765 7200
Fax: 020 8765 7211
Website: www.ageconcern.org.uk
Researches into the needs of older people and is involved in policy making. Publishes many books and has useful factsheets on a wide range of issues from benefits to care, and provides services via local branches.

Age Concern Scotland
113 Rose Street
Edinburgh EH2 3DT
Help Line: 0800 009966
Tel: 0131 220 3345
Fax: 0131 220 2779
Website: www.ageconcernscotland.org.uk
Supplies information sheets and local support groups offering a variety of services to the elderly.

AREMCO
Grove House
Lenham
Kent ME17 2PX
Tel: 01622 858502
Fax: 01622 850532
Suppliers of a variety of equipment, aids and tools for people with disabilities; protective headgear, bed-leaving alarms and swivel seats for cars etc.

Artsline
54 Chalton Street
London NW1 1HS
Tel: 020 7388 2227
Fax: 020 7383 2653
Website: www.artsline.org.uk
Offers information on arts and entertainments venues which have disabled access for people with disabilities.

Assistance Travel Service Ltd
1 Tank Lane
Purfleet RM19 1TA
Tel: 01708 863198
Fax: 01708 860514
Website: aatstravel@aol.com
Specializes in supporting people on holidays throughout the UK and the world who need nursing or a range of other support services.

Association of Community Health Councils for England & Wales
Earlsmead House
30 Drayton Park
London N5 1PB
Tel: 020 7609 8405
Fax: 020 7700 1152
Website: www.achcew.org.uk
Headquarters for local community health councils who represent the needs of the patient.

Association of Disabled Professionals
BCM ADP
London WC1N 3XX
Tel: 020 8778 5008
Fax: 0239 224 1420
Website: www.adp.org.uk
Promotes education, rehabilitation, training and employment opportunities available to professional people with disabilities. Offers advice, information and peer support to disabled people. Also funds research.

Association of Professional Music Therapists
26 Hamlyn Road
Glastonbury BA6 8HT
Tel: 01458 834919
Fax: 01458 834919
Website: www.apmt.org.uk
Body setting standards of training and practice among professional music therapists. Can refer to local music therapists.

Association of Reflexologists
27 Old Gloucester Street
London WC1N 3XX
Tel: 0870 567 3320
Fax: 01989 567676
Website: www.aor.org.uk
Accreditation body offering lists of practitioners and training courses for reflexology.

BBC Audio Books
St James House
The Square
Lower Bristol Road
Bath BA2 3SB
Tel: 01225 878000
Fax: 01225 448005
Website: www.audiobookcollection.com
www.largeprintdirect.co.uk
Books in large print and audio tapes for sale. Mail order only.

Benefits Enquiry Line (BEL) (for people with disabilities)
Help Line: 0800 882200
Freephone: N. Ireland 0800 220674
Minicom: 0800 243355
Website: www.dwp.gov.uk
Government agency giving information and advice on sickness and disability benefits for people with disabilities and their carers.

British Acupuncture Council
63 Jeddo Road
London W12 9HQ
Tel: 020 8735 0400
Fax: 020 8735 0404
Website: www.acupuncture.org.uk
Professional body offering lists of qualified acupuncture therapists.

British Association for Counselling and Psychotherapy
1 Regent Place
Rugby CV21 2PJ
Helpline: 0870 443 5252
Tel: 01788 550899
Fax: 0870 443 5160
Website: www.bacp.co.uk
Professional services organization and directory of professional counsellors. Offers lists of all levels of counsellors and can refer to specialist counselling services.

British Association of Cricketers with Disabilities
26 Kelthorpe Close
Stamford PE9 3RS
Tel: 01780 720496
Fax: 01780 721443
Organizes cricket for people with physical or learning disabilities. Can refer to local groups.

British Complementary Medicine Association
PO Box 5122
Bournemouth BH8 OWG
Tel/Fax: 0845 345 5977
Website: www.bcma.co.uk
Multitherapy umbrella body representing organizations, clinics, colleges and independent schools, and acting as the voice of complementary medicine.

British Council of Disabled People
Litchurch Plaza
Litchurch Lane
Derby DE24 8AA
Tel: 01332 295551
Fax: 01332 295580
Minicom: 01332 295581
Website: www.bcodp.org.uk
Offers information on human and civil rights and support for organizations of disabled people.

British Herbal Medicine Association
1 Wickham Road
Boscombe
Bournemouth BH7 6JX
Tel: 01202 433691
Fax: 01202 417079
Website: www.bhma.info
Offers information, encourages research and promotes high quality standards. Advises members on legalities for importers, vets advertisements and defends the right of the public to choose herbal medicines and be able to obtain them freely.

British Holistic Medical Association
59 Lansdowne Place
Hove BN3 1FL
Tel: 01273 725951
Fax: 01273 725951
Website: www.bhma.org
Promotes awareness of the holistic approach to health among practitioners and the public through publications, self-help tapes, conferences and a network of local groups.

British Homeopathic Association
15 Clerkenwell Close
London EC1R 0AA
Tel: 020 7566 7800
Fax: 020 7566 7815
Website: www.trusthomeopathy.org
Professional body offering lists of qualified homeopathic practitioners.

British Medical Acupuncture Society
12 Marbury House
Higher Whitley
Warrington WA4 4QW
Tel: 01925 730727
Fax: 01925 730492
Website: www.medical-acupuncture.co.uk
Professional body offering training to doctors and list of accredited acupuncture practitioners.

British Red Cross Society
9 Grosvenor Crescent
London SW1X 7EJ
Tel: 020 7235 5454
Fax: 020 7245 6315
Website: www.redcross.org.uk
Gives skilled and impartial care to people in need and crisis in their own homes, the community, at home and abroad, in peace and in war. Refers to local branches.

British Reflexology Association (BRA)
Monks Orchard
Whitbourne
Worcester WR6 5RB
Tel: 01886 821207
Fax: 01886 822017
Website: www.britreflex.co.uk
Professional body offering training and list of accredited members.

**British Society for Disability
and Oral Health**
Dental Special Needs Unit
Chorley District General Hospital
Preston Road
Chorley PR7 1PP
Tel: 012572 45664
Website: www.bsdh.org.uk
*NHS dental service for people with disabilities
with dental problems.*

**British Sports Association for
the Disabled – Northern Ireland**
Sports Council
House of Sport
Upper Malone Road
Belfast, BT9 5LA
Tel: 01232 381222

British Wheel of Yoga
25 Jermyn Street
Sleaford NG34 7RU
Tel: 01529 306851
Fax: 01529 303233
Website: www.bwy.org.uk
*Professional body offering lists of qualified
yoga therapists.*

Carers North of England
23 New Mount Street,
Manchester.
M4 4DE
Tel: 0161 953 4233
Fax: 0161 953 4092
*Campaigns on behalf of, and offers
information and support to, all people who
have to care for others due to medical or other
problems in the north of England.*

Carers Northern Ireland
58 Howard Street,
Belfast.
BT1 6PJ
Tel: 028 9043 9843
Fax: 028 9043 9299
*Campaigns on behalf of, and offers
information and support to, all people who
have to care for others due to medical or other
problems in Northern Ireland.*

Carers Scotland
91 Mitchell Street
Glasgow G1 3LN
Helpline: 0808 808 7777
Tel: 0141 221 9141
Fax: 0141 221 9140
Website: www.carersonline.org.uk
*Campaigns on behalf of, and offers
information and support to, all people who
have to care for others due to medical or other
problems in Scotland.*

Carers UK
20–25 Glasshouse Yard
London EC1A 4JT
Helpline: 0808 808 7777
Tel: 020 7490 8818
Fax: 020 7490 8824
Website: www.carersonline.org.uk
*Offers information and support to all people
who are unpaid carers, looking after others
with medical or other problems in UK.*

Carers Wales
River House,
Ynysbridge Court,
Gwaelod y Garth,
Cardiff
CF15 9SS
Tel: 029 2081 1370
Fax: 029 2081 1575
*Campaigns on behalf of, and offers
information and support to, all people who
have to care for others due to medical or other
problemsin Wales.*

**Chartwell Insurance & Disabled Drivers
Insurance Bureau**
292–294 Hale Lane
Edgware HA8 8NP
Tel: 020 8958 0900
Fax: 020 8958 3220
Website: www.chartwellinsurance.co.uk
*Gives information and advice on vehicle and
power chair insurance with particular emphasis
on drivers with disabilities. Also covers
household, travel and commercial insurance.*

Chester-Care/Homecraft
Sidings Road
Low Moor Estate
Kirkby-in-Ashfield NG17 7QX
Helpline: 01623 757555
Tel: 01623 757955
Fax: 01623 755585
Website: www.homecraftability1.com
*Manufactures and distributes a variety of
rehabilitation aids for walking including
bathroom and toileting range for people with
disabilities. Mail order available.*

**Citizen Advocacy Information
and Training (CAIT)**
162 Lea Valley Technopark
Ashley Road
Tottenham Hale
London N17 9LN
Tel: 020 8880 4545
Fax: 020 8880 4113
Website: www.citizenadvocacy.org.uk
*Promotes, supports and offers free, friendly
advocacy by one citizen to another.*

**Citizens Advice
(formerly Citizens Advice Bureau)**
Myddleton House
115–123 Pentonville Road
London N1 9LZ
Helpline: 0870 750 9000
Tel: 020 7833 2181
Fax: 020 7833 4371
Website: www.citizensadvice.org.uk
*Headquarters of national charity offering a
wide variety of practical, financial and legal
advice. Network of local branches throughout
the UK listed in phone books and in Yellow
Pages under Counselling and Advice.*

Citizens Advice Scotland
Spectrum House
2 Powderhall Road
Edinburgh EH7 4GB
Tel: 0131 550 1000
Fax: 0131 550 1001
Website: www.cas.org.uk
*Provide details of local Citizens Advice
bureaux, which are also available in local
telephone directories.*

Community Health Council
The address and telephone number of
your local CHC will be in the Phone Book
and in Yellow Pages.
Website: www.achcew.org.uk
*Statutory information service offering advice
to users of the National Health Service. Local
branches.*

Community Service Volunteers
237 Pentonville Road
London N1 9NJ
Tel: 020 7278 6601
Fax: 020 7833 0149
Website: www.csv.org.uk
*Encourages people through training and
support to take action in their communities.
Provides volunteers to work full time in social
care placements for periods of 4–12 months.*

Compassionate Friends
53 North Street
Bedminster
Bristol BS3 1EN
Helpline: 0117 953 9639
Tel: 0117 966 5202
Fax: 0117 914 4368
Website: www.tcf.org.uk
*Befrienders who offer information and
support to parents, siblings and close family
members who have lost a child. Support
groups locally.*

Continence Foundation
307 Hatton Square
16 Baldwins Gardens
London EC1N 7RJ
Helpline: 0845 345 0165
Tel: 020 7404 6875
Fax: 020 7404 6876
Website: www.continence-foundation.org.uk
*Offers information and support for people
with bladder and/or bowel problems. Has
lists of regional specialists.*

Crossroads: Caring for Carers
10 Regent Place
Rugby CV21 2PN
Tel: 01788 573653
Fax: 01788 565498
Wales: 02920 222282
Website: www.crossroads.org.uk
Supports and delivers high quality services for
carers and people with care needs via its local
branches. Additional helplines:

Crossroads Scotland
24 George Square
Glasgow G2 1EG
Tel: 0141 226 3793
Fax: 0141 221 7130
Website: www.crossroads-scotland.co.uk
Information leaflets on respite care and
support for carers within own homes, for any
age, disability and sickness. Local branches.

Cruse Bereavement Care
Cruse House
126 Sheen Road
Richmond TW9 1UR
Helpline: 0870 167 1677
Tel: 020 8940 4818
Fax: 020 8940 7638
Website: www.crusebereavementcare.org.uk
Offers information, practical advice, sells
literature and has local branches which can
provide 1 to 1 counselling to people who have
been bereaved. Training in bereavement
counselling for professionals.

DIAL UK
St Catherines
Tickhill Road
Balby
Doncaster DN4 8QN
Tel: 01302 310123
Fax: 01302 310404
Website: www.dialuk.org.uk
Offers advice on all aspects of disability.

Dialability
Oxford Centre for Enablement
Windmill Road
Headington OX3 7LD
Tel: 01865 763600
Fax: 01865 764730
Email: helpline@dialability.org.uk
Offers information and advice to people with
disabilities, carers and professionals on a
variety of leisure and recreation issues,
holidays, sports and adult education. Also has
a showroom where equipment to aid people
with disabilities can be viewed.

Disabilities Trust
First Floor
32 Market Place
Burgess Hill RH15 9NP
Tel: 01444 239123
Fax: 01444 244978
Website: www.disabilities-trust.org.uk
Offers care and long term accommodation for
people with autism, acquired brain injury and
physical disabilities at 18 centres across
England.

Disability Alliance
Universal House
88–94 Wentworth Street
London E1 7SA
Helpline: 020 7247 8763
Tel: 020 7247 8776
Fax: 020 7247 8765
Website: www.disabilityalliance.org
Offers information on benefits through
publications (Disability Rights Handbook),
free briefing sheets, rights advice line and
training. Campaigns for improvements to the
social security system.

Disability Equipment Register
4 Chatterton Road
Yate
Bristol BS37 4BJ
Tel: 01454 318818
Fax: 01454 883870
Website: www.disabilityequipment.org.uk
Nationwide service, via magazine, to buy and
sell used disability equipment.

Disability Information Trust
Mary Marlborough Centre
Nuffield Orthopaedic Centre
Headington
Oxford OX3 7LD
Tel: 01865 227592

Disability Law Service
39–45 Cavell Street
London E1 2BP
Tel: 020 7791 9800
Fax: 020 7791 9802
*Provides free legal advice for people with
disabilities.*

Disability Now
(campaigning newspaper)
Editorial Department
6 Market Road
London N7 9PW
Tel: 020 7619 7323
Fax: 020 7619 7331
Minicom: 020 7619 7332
Website: www.disabilitynow.org.uk
*Newspaper publishing news and views for and
about people with disabilities. Available nation-
wide via newsagents and by subscription.*

Disability Rights Commission
FREEPOST
MID 02164
Stratford upon Avon CV37 9BR
Tel: 08457 622633
Fax: 08457 778878
Website: www.drc-gb.org
*Government-sponsored centre offering
publications and up-to-date information on
the Disability Discrimination Act. Special
team of advisers can help with problems of
discrimination at work.*

Disability Sport England
Solecast House
13/27 Brunswick Place
London N1 6DX
Tel: 020 7490 4919
*Provides opportunities for people of all ages
with disabilities to take part in sport. Has
regional offices.*

Disability Sports Northern Ireland
House of Sport
Upper Malone Road
Belfast BT9 5LA
Tel: 02890 381222
Fax: 02890 682757
Website: www.sportni.com
*Administrative headquarters for sport in
Northern Ireland catering for able and
disabled people; refers to local organizations.*

Disability Wales/Anabledd Cymru
Wernddu Court
Caerphilly Business Park
Van Road
Mid Glamorgan CF83 3ED
Helpline: 0800 731 6282
Tel: 0292 088 7325
Fax: 0292 088 8702
Website: www.dwac.demon.co.uk
*Promotes rights, inclusion, equality and
support of all disabled people in Wales. Refers
to local branches.*

Disabled Access to Technology
Association
Neville House
Neville Road
Bradford BD4 8TU
Tel: 01274 370019
Fax: 01274 723861
Website: www.databradford.org
*Trains people with disabilities to enable them
to get back to work.*

Disabled Christians Fellowship
Global House
Ashley Avenue
Epsom KT18 5AD
Tel: 01372 737046
Fax: 01372 737040
Minicom: 01372 737041
Website: www.throughtheroof.org
*Fellowship by correspondence, cassettes, local
branches, holidays, youth section, local
workshop and day centre.*

Disabled Drivers Association, National Headquarters
Ashwelthorpe
Norwich NR16 1EX
Tel: 0870 770 3333
Fax: 01508 488173
Website: www.dda.org.uk
Self-help association offering information and advice and aiming for independence through mobility.

Disabled Drivers Motor Club
Cottingham Way
Thrapston
Northants NN14 4PL
Tel: 01832 734724
Fax: 01832 733816
Website: www.ddmc.org.uk
Offers information service to disabled drivers about ferries, airports and insurance. Subscription for monthly magazine.

Disabled Living Centres Council
Redbank House
4 St Chads Street
Cheetham
Manchester M8 8QA
Tel: 0161 834 1044
Fax: 0161 839 0802
Textphone: 0161 839 0885
Website: www.dlcc.org.uk
Coordinates work of Disabled Living Centres UK wide. Offers lists of centres and the different services they provide.

Disabled Living Foundation
380–384 Harrow Road
London W9 2HU
Helpline: 0845 130 9177
Tel: 020 7289 6111
Fax: 020 7266 2922
Textphone: (Minicom): 020 7432 8009
Website: www.dlf.org.uk
Provides information to disabled and older people on all kinds of equipment in order to promote their indepence and quality of life.

Disabled Motorists Federation
145 Knoulberry Road
Blackfell
Washington NE37 1JN
Tel: 0191 416 3172
Fax: 0191 416 3172
Self-help organization offering information to drivers with disabilities and campaigning on their behalf for better motoring and public transport facilities. Arranges concessions for ferry bookings. Local groups.

Disablement Income Group Scotland
5 Quayside Street
Edinburgh EH6 6EJ
Tel: 0131 555 2811
Fax: 0131 554 7076
Promotes the financial welfare of disabled people with advice service on rights and benefits. Membership (optional) available for £5.

DVLA (Drivers and Vehicles Licensing Authority
Medical Branch
Longview Road
Morriston
Swansea SA99 1TU
Helpline: 0870 600 0301
Tel: 0870 240 0009
Fax: 01792 783779
Website: www.dvla.gov.uk
Government office offering advice to drivers with medical conditions.

Employment Opportunities for People with Disabilities
123 Minories
London EC3N 1NT
Tel: 020 7481 2727
Fax: 020 7481 9797
Website: www.opportunities.org.uk
Helps people with disabilities find and retain employment through training, mock interviews, assessment, graduate scheme and support during placements. Regional centres offer training on disability awareness to employers.

Equal Opportunities Commission
Arndale House
Arndale Centre
Manchester M4 3EQ
Tel: 0845 601 5901
Fax: 0161 838 1733
Website: www.eoc.org.uk
*Investigates cases of sex discrimination
and equal pay issues. Offers a range of
information, freely available on the website.*

FABB Scotland
5a Warriston Road
Edinburgh EH3 5LQ
Tel: 0131 558 9912
*Headquarters in Scotland for network of local
groups who arrange integrated projects to
bring disabled and able-bodied people together.*

Family Fund Trust
PO Box 50
York YO1 9ZX
Helpline: 0845 130 4542
Tel: 01904 621115
Fax: 01904 652625
Website: www.familyfundtrust.org.uk
*Offers information and grants for items such
as bedding, washing machines, holidays or
driving lessons to families in the UK with
children of up to 16 years with special care
needs. Apply direct.*

Family Service Units
207 Old Marylebone Road
London NW1 5QP
Tel: 020 7402 5175
Fax: 020 7724 1829
Website: www.fsu.org.uk
*Offers a range of support to children and
families disadvantaged by poverty and at risk
of social exclusion.*

Family Welfare Association
501–505 Kingsland Road
London E8 4AU
Tel: 020 7254 6251
Fax: 020 7249 5443
Website: www.fwa.org.uk
*Runs family drop-in centres and mental
health residential homes. Students may apply
for education grants direct; s.a.e. requested.
Only accepts requests for welfare grants from
professionals in writing.*

FES Team
Medical Physics Department
Salisbury District Hospital
Salisbury SP2 8BJ
Tel: 01722 336262 (ext. 4065)

Foundation for Assistive Technology
12 City Forum
250 City Road
London EC1V 8AF
Tel: 020 7253 3303
Fax: 020 7253 5990
Website: www.fastuk.org
*Information resource and exchange platform
for new development projects in aids for
people with disabilities. Researches into new
equipment to aid people with disabilities.*

Foundations
Bleaklow House
Howard Town Mill
Glossop SK13 8HT
Tel: 01457 891909
Fax: 01457 869361
Website: www.foundations.uk.com
*Coordinating body for Home Improvement
Agencies throughout England. These offer free
help to older or disabled home owners and
private sector tenants on low incomes to
repair, improve or adapt premises to enable
them to stay in their own homes.*

General Osteopathic Council
Osteopathy House
176 Tower Bridge Road
London SE1 3LU
Tel: 020 7357 6655
Fax: 020 7357 0011
Website: www.osteopathy.org.uk
Regulatory body that offers information to
the public and lists of accredited osteopaths.

Gingerbread (organization for lone parent
families)
7 Sovereign Court
Sovereign Close
London E1W 3HW
Helpline: 0800 018 4318
Tel: 020 7488 9300
Fax: 020 7488 9333
Website: www.gingerbread.org.uk
National network of self-help groups for lone
parents and children. Has publications and
advice line covering legal, benefits and
emotional issues.

Health Development Agency
Trevelyan House
30 Great Peter Street
London SW1P 2HW
Helpline: 0800 555777
Website: www.hda-online.org.uk
Formerly Health Education Authority; now
only deals with research. Publications on
health matters can be ordered via helpline.

Help for Health Trust
Highcroft
Romsey Road
Winchester SO22 5DH
Tel: 01962 849100
Fax: 01962 849079
Website: www.hfht.org
The Trust aims to enable people to become
active partners in their own health care by
improving the provision of quality health
information. Databases Helpbox and NHS
A–Z available via website.

Holiday Care
7th Floor
Sunley House
4 Bedford Park
Croydon CR0 2AP
Tel: 0845 124 9971
Fax: 0845 124 9972
Website: www.holidaycare.org.uk
Provides holiday advice on venues and tour
operators for people with special needs.

Holidays (Help the Handicapped – 3H
Fund)
147a Camden Road
Tunbridge Wells TN1 2RA
Tel: 01892 547474
Fax: 01892 524703
Website: www.3hfund.org.uk
Subsidized group holidays for physically
disabled children and adults with volunteer
carers, offering respite for regular carers.
Grants to low income families with physically
or mentally disabled dependents to have a
modest UK holiday. Apply direct.

Horticulture for All
c/o The Institute of Horticulture
14–15 Belgrave Square
London SW1X 8PS
Prints publications on a wide variety of
subjects concerning horticulture for people
with disabilities. Information on toxic plants,
polluted areas and qualifications. Organizes
conferences on horticulture for people with
disabilities.

Huntleigh Health Care
310–312 Dallow Road
Luton LU1 1TD
Tel: 01582 413104
Fax: 01582 459100
Website: www.huntleigh-healthcare.com
Manufacturers of medical equipment and
pressure-relieving garments for mattresses.
Available via mail order.

Incontact – Action on Incontinence
United House
North Road
London N7 9DP
Tel: 020 7700 3246
Fax: 020 7700 3249
Website: www.incontact.org
*Information and help via local support and
user groups for people with bladder and bowel
problems.*

Independent Living Alternatives
Trafalgar House
Grenville Place
London NW7 3SA
Tel: 020 8906 9265
Fax: 020 8906 9265
Website: www.i-l-a.fsnet.co.uk
*Advice on how to obtain cash entitlement
from benefit agencies by direct payment in
lieu of meals on wheels or home help from
local authorities.*

Independent Living Fund
PO Box 7525
Nottingham NG2 4ZT
Tel: 0845 601 8815
Fax: 0115 945 0948
Website: www.ilf.org.uk
*Offers financial assistance in the UK for
buying personal and/or domestic care.
Applicants must already be receiving the
highest care allowance and at least £200.
care package from Social Services. Referral
via Social Services.*

Institute for Complementary Medicine
PO Box 194
London SE16 7QZ
Tel: 020 7237 5165
Fax: 020 7237 5175
Website: www.icmedicine.co.uk
*Umbrella group for complementary medicine
organizations. Offers informed, safe choice
to public, British register of practitioners
and refers to accredited training courses.
S.a.e. requested for information.*

J. D. Williams (Special Collection)
53 Dale Street
Manchester M60 6ES
Tel: 0161 238 2000
Fax: 0161 238 2025
Website: www.jdwilliams.co.uk
*A mail order catalogue of fashion clothing
and footwear available in large sizes.*

John Grooms
50 Scrutton Street
London EC2A 4XQ
Tel: 020 7452 2000
Fax: 020 7452 2001
Website: www.johngrooms.org.uk
*Charity providing a range of residential care,
housing, holidays and work across the UK.*

Joolys Joint
Website: www.mswsebpals.org
*A free American website for people with MS
supporting each other.*

Jubilee Sailing Trust
www.jst.co.uk

Keep Able Ltd
Sterling Park
Pedmore Road
Brierley Hill DY5 1TB
Tel: 01384 484544
Fax: 01384 480802
Website: www.keepable.co.uk
*Distributors of equipment and aids for the
elderly and less able. Home assessments for
stairlifts, wheelchairs etc. Available via mail
order. Some regional stores.*

Law Centres Federation
Duchess House
18–19 Warren Street
London W1T 5LR
Tel: 020 7387 8570
Fax: 020 7387 8368
Website: www.lawcentres.org.uk
*Headquarters of national law centres. Can
refer to local law centres and website for free
information and advice.*

Law Society
114 Chancery Lane
London WC2A 1PL
Tel: 020 7320 5793
Fax: 020 7831 0170
Website: www.gsdnet.org.uk
Offers help and support to law students and solicitors with disabilities.

Leonard Cheshire
30 Millbank
London SW1P 4QD
Tel: 020 7802 8200
Fax: 020 7802 8250
Website: www.leonard-cheshire.org
Offers care, support and a wide range of information for disabled people between 18 and 65 years in the UK and worldwide to encourage independent living. Respite and residential homes, holidays and rehabilitation.

Liberty (The National Council for Civil Liberties)
21 Tabard Street
London SE1 4LA
Helpline: 020 7378 8659
Tel: 020 7403 3888
Fax: 020 7407 5354
Website: www.liberty-human-rights.org.uk
Pressure group which protects and extends human rights and civil liberties. Offers information and free legal advice helpline.

Listening Books
12 Lant Street
London SE1 1QH
Tel: 020 7407 9417
Fax: 020 7403 1377
Website: www.listening-books.org.uk
Provides audio books, for both pleasure and learning, on tape for adults and children suitable for anyone who cannot hold a book, turn pages or read in the usual way. Subscription for lending library of tapes by mail order.

Long-Term Medical Conditions Alliance (LMCA)
c/o Unit 212
16 Baldwins Gardens
London EC1N 7RJ
Tel: 020 7813 3637
Fax: 020 7813 3640
Website: www.lmca.org.uk
Campaigns to improve the quality of life of people with long-term medical conditions.

Medic-Alert Foundation
1 Bridge Wharf
156 Caledonian Road
London N1 9UU
Helpline: 0800 581420
Tel: 020 7833 3034
Fax: 020 7278 0647
Website: www.medicalert.org.uk
A life-saving body-worn identification system for people with hidden medical conditions. 24-hour emergency telephone number. Offers selection of jewellery with internationally recognized medical symbol.

Mobility Advice & Vehicle Information Service (MAVIS)
O Wing
Macadam Avenue
Old Wokingham Road
Crowthorne RG45 6XD
Tel: 01344 661000
Fax: 01344 661066
Website: www.mobility-unit.dft.gov.uk
Government department offering driving and vehicle assessment to people with disabilities. Can advise on vehicle adaptations for both drivers and passengers.

Mobility Information Service and Disabled Motorists Club
National Mobility Centre
Unit B1 Greenwood Court
Cartmel Drive
Shrewsbury SY1 3TB
Tel: 01743 463072
Fax: 01743 463065
Website: www.mis.org.uk
Information on mobility. Driving assessment for disabled drivers at regional centres.

Motability
Goodman House
Station Approach
Harlow CM20 2ET
Tel: 01279 635666
Fax: 01279 632000
Minicom: 01279 632273
Website: www.motability.co.uk
Advises people with disabilities about powered wheelchairs, scooters, new and used cars, how to adapt them to their needs and obtain funding via the Mobility Scheme.

**National Centre
for Independent Living**
250 Kennington Lane
London SE11 5RD
Tel: 020 7587 1663
Fax: 020 7582 2469
Website: www.ncil.org.uk
Provides information, consultancy and training on personal assistance and direct payments. Advice for obtaining payment from the benefits system to enable people to buy private personal care instead of receiving it via the local authority.

National Childbirth Trust
Alexandra House
Oldham Terrace
London W3 6NH
Helpline: 08704 448708
Tel: 08704 448707
Fax: 08707 703237
Website: www.nctpregnancyandbabycare.com
Parent-to-parent support via local groups. Antenatal classes and breastfeeding counselling by trained teachers. Breastfeeding counselling helpline available 8am–10pm. Information, pre- and postnatal classes.

National Gardens Scheme
Hatchlands Park
East Clandon
Guildford GU4 7RT
Tel: 01483 211535
Fax: 01483 211537
Website: www.ngs.org.uk
Provides list of privately owned gardens of quality, character and interest which, for a donation to charity, are open to the public at certain times of year.

**National Institute
of Medical Herbalists**
56 Longbrook Street
Exeter EX4 6AH
Tel: 01392 426022
Fax: 01392 498963
Website: www.nimh.org.uk
Professional body representing qualified, practising medical herbalists. Offers lists of accredited medical herbalists. S.a.e. requested.

Open University (OU)
Disability Advisory Services
Disabled Students Services Section
Walton Hall
Milton Keynes MK7 6AA
Tel: 01908 652255
Fax: 01908 659956
Website: www.open.ac.uk
Offers advice to people who wish to study accredited educational courses at home. Provides materials in alternative format, e.g. tapes, CDs.

Oxford Centre for Enablement
Windmill Road
Headington OX3 7LD
Tel: 01865 227600
Website: www.rivermeadrehabilitation.nhs/
A rehabilitation centre for people recovering from head injuries and strokes. Also offers day respite care for people with other long term illnesses such as MS.

Partially Sighted Society
PO Box 322
Doncaster DN1 2XA
Tel: 01302 323132
Fax: 01302 368998
Email: info@partsight.org.uk
Assists visually impaired people to make the
best use of their remaining vision with a
range of useful publications and equipment
available by mail order.

Patients Association
PO Box 935
Harrow HA1 3YJ
Helpline: 0845 608 4455
Tel: 020 8423 9111
Fax: 020 8423 9119
Website: www.patients-association.com
Provides advice on patients' rights. Leaflets
and directory of self-help groups available.

Pensions Advisory Service (OPAS)
11 Belgrave Road
London SW1V 1RB
Tel: 08456 012923
Fax: 020 7233 8016
Website: www.opas.org.uk
Free help to people with problems with
occupational, personal and stakeholder
pensions. State pensions are not dealt with
but referred appropriately.

PHAB
Summit House
50 Wandle Road
Croydon CR0 1DF
Tel: 020 8667 9443
Fax: 020 8681 1399
Website: www.phabengland.org.uk
Headquarters for a national network of local
clubs who arrange integrated projects to bring
disabled and able-bodied people together.

PHAB Scotland *see* **FABB Scotland**

PHAB Wales
2nd Floor
St David's House
Wood Street
Cardiff CF1 1ES
Tel: 01222 223677
Website: www.phabwales.org.uk
Headquarters in Wales for network of local
groups who arrange integrated projects to
bring disabled and able-bodied people together.

Planetamber
www.planetamber/resources/207.html
Perhaps one of the most comprehensive
listings of websites giving information and
advice for the UK and elsewhere: the site is
described as a global health and disability
resource centre. Contains over 25 UK sites
and many more overseas catering for a wide
range of disabilities and health problems, and
offering a wide range of support services.

Queen Elizabeth Foundation
for Disabled People
Leatherhead Court
Woodlands Road
Leatherhead KT22 0BN
Tel: 01372 841100
Fax: 01372 844072
Website: www.qefd.org
Provides information, demonstrations,
assessment and training on outdoor mobility
for professionals and people with disabilities.

RADAR
(Royal Association for Disability
& Rehabilitation)
12 City Forum
250 City Road
London EC1V 8AF
Tel: 020 7250 3222
Fax: 020 7250 0212
Minicom: 020 7250 4119
Website: www.radar.org.uk
Campaigns to improve rights and care of
disabled people. Offers advice on every aspect
of living with a disability and refers to other
agencies for training and rehabilitation.

Rail Unit for Disabled Passengers Switchboard
Helpline: 08700 005151
Queries about travelling within the UK rail network referred to appropriate areas for advice. Enquirers must provide specific details of destination in order to be referred to appropriate railway company.

Relate (Marriage Guidance)
Herbert Gray College
Little Church Street
Rugby CV21 3AP
Helpline: 0845 130 4010
Tel: 01788 573241
Fax: 01788 535007
Website: www.relate.org.uk
Offers relationship counselling via local branches. Relate publications on health, sexual, self-esteem, depression, bereavement and re-marriage issues available from bookshops, libraries or via website.

REMAP
Hazeldene
Ightham
Sevenoaks TN15 9AD
Tel: 01732 883818
Tel: 01737 355388 (*regional contacts – London and South East*)
Tel: 0121 475 6919 (*Midlands and Wales*)
Tel: 01485 542412 (*East*)
Tel: 01732 883818 (*North East & West*)
Tel: 01566 775304 (*South West*)
Tel: 01294 832566 (*Scotland*)
Tel: 01232 791991 (*Northern Ireland*)
Website: www.remap.org.uk
Makes or adapts aids, when not commercially available, for people with disabilities at no charge to the disabled person. Local branches.

REMPLOY
Stonecourt
Siskin Drive
Coventry CV3 4FJ
Tel: 02476 515800
Fax: 02476 515860
Website: www.remploy.co.uk
Finds employment for people with disabilities in own factories throughout the UK and elsewhere. Offers assessment at work; has training facilities in Remploy learning centres.

Riding for the Disabled Association
Lavinia Norfolk House
Avenue R,
Stoneleigh Park
Kenilworth CV8 2LY
Tel: 0247 669 6510
Fax: 0247 669 6532
Website: www.riding-for-disabled.org.uk
Provides the opportunity of riding and carriage driving to people of all ages with disabilities.

Royal London Homeopathic Hospital
Great Ormond Street
London WC1N 3HR
Tel: 020 7837 8833
NHS Hospital which treats patients with homeopathic medicines. Only accepts referrals from general practitioners. (Temporarily housed at Greenwell Street, London W1W 5BP during refurbishment of Hospital in Great Ormond Street.)

Scottish Disability Sport
Fife Sport Institute
Viewfield Road
Glenrothes KY6 2RB
Tel: 01592 415700
Fax: 01592 415710
Website: www.scottishdisabilitysport.com
Organizes sports and competition events for people with disabilities. Refers to local branches.

Scottish Sports Association for People with a Disability (SSAD)
Fife Institute PRE
Viewfield Road
Glenrothes KY6 2RB
Tel: 01592 415700

Scouts Holiday Homes Trust
Gilwell Park
Bury Road
Chingford E4 7QW
Tel: 020 8433 7290
Fax: 020 8433 7103
Website:
www.scoutbase.org.uk-hq-info/holidayhomes
Offers low cost, self-catering holidays on fully commercial holiday parks for disabled and disadvantaged people. No scouting connection necessary.

Sequal Trust
3 Ploughmans Corner
Wharf Road
Ellesmere SY12 0EJ
Tel: 01691 624222
Fax: 01691 624222
Website: www.the-sequal-trust.org.uk
Fundraising charity which helps provide and then maintain communication aids for people disabled with speech, movement or learning difficulties.

Shaftesbury Society
16 Kingston Road
London SW19 1JZ
Tel: 020 8239 5555
Fax: 020 8239 5580
Website: www.shaftesburysoc.org.uk
Christian organization provides residential centres, schools, colleges and holiday centres for disabled people of all religious faiths. Has prayer line.

Shirley Price Aromatherapy
Essentia House
Upper Bond Street
Hinckley LE10 1RS
Tel: 01455 615466
Fax: 01455 615054
Website: www.shirleyprice.com
Sources and supplies natural pure essential oils and carriers for aromatherapy. International college training to professional standards and lists of local therapists accredited by IFPA (International Federation of Prof. Aromatherapists) Mail order.

SKILL (National Bureau for Students with Disabilities)
Chapter House
18–20 Crucifix Lane
London SE1 3JW
Helpline: 0800 328 5050
Tel: 020 7450 0620
Fax: 020 7450 0650
Textline: 0800 068 2422
Website: www.skill.org.uk
Provides information, advice and support for students with disabilities 16 years and over on funding, training and employment.

Snowden Award Scheme
22 City Business Centre
6 Brighton Road
Horsham RH13 5BB
Tel: 01403 211252
Fax: 01403 271553
Website: www.snowdenawardscheme.org.uk
Bursaries to help physically disabled students with the additional costs of further and higher education or training. Apply direct.

SPOD (Association to aid the Sexual & Personal Relationships of People with a Disability)
286 Camden Road
London N7 0BJ
Helpline: 020 7607 9191
Tel: 020 7607 8851
Fax: 020 7700 0236
Website: www.spod-uk.org
Provides information and advice on the problems in sex and personal relationships that disability can cause.

Sports Council for Wales
Sophia Gardens
Cardiff CF1 9SW
Tel: 02920 300500
Fax: 02920 300600
Website: www.sports-councilwales.co.uk
Headquarters for national network of local clubs who arrange integrated projects to bring disabled and able-bodied people together. Promotes sport in Wales and distributes lottery funding. Supports Paralympic athletes.

SSAFA Forces Help
Special Needs Advisor
19 Queen Elizabeth Street
London SE1 2LP
Tel: 020 7403 8783
Fax: 020 7403 8815
Website: www.ssafa.org.uk
National charity offering information, advice and financial aid to serving and ex-servicemen and women and their families who are in need.

Talking Newspapers Association UK
National Recording Centre
Browning Road
Heathfield TN21 8DB
Tel: 01435 866102
Fax: 01435 865422
Website: www.tnauk.org.uk
Lists 200 national newspapers and magazines on tape, computer, CD-ROM and email for loan to visually impaired, blind and physically disabled people. Annual subscription.

Telework Association
WREN Telecottage
Stoneleigh Park
Kenilworth CV8 2RR
Helpline: 0800 616008
Tel: 02476 696986
Fax: 02476 696538
Website: www.telework.org.uk
Information handbook on legal and practical aspects of setting up a home business.

Thrive
The Geoffrey Udall Centre
Trunkwell Park
Beach Hill
Reading RG7 2AT
Tel: 0118 988 5688
An organization providing information and advice on gardening with a disability. It produces a number of leaflets and has a quarterly magazine.

Tripscope
The Vassal Centre
Gill Avenue
Bristol BS16 2QQ
Tel: 08457 585641
Fax: 01179 397736
Website: www.tripscope.org.uk
Provides comprehensive information for elderly and disabled people on all aspects of travelling within the UK and abroad.

Ulverscroft Large Print Books
1 The Green
Bradgate Road
Anstey LE7 7FU
Tel: 0116 236 4325
Fax: 0116 234 020 5
Website: www.ulverscroft.co.uk
Publishes large print books which are available at libraries and via mailorder.

Winged Fellowship Trust
Angel House
20–32 Pentonville Road
LondonN1 9XD
Tel: 020 7833 2594
Fax: 020 7278 0370
Website: www.wft.org.uk
*Provides holidays at their own UK centres
and overseas and respite care for people with
severe physical disabilities by providing
volunteer carers. Also arranges holidays for
people with dementia/Alzheimer's disease
and their own carers.*

Yoga for Health Foundation
Ickwell Bury
Biggleswade SG18 9EF
Tel: 01767 627271
Fax: 01767 627266
Website: www.yogaforhealthfoundation.co.uk
*Offers teacher training for remedial yoga at
their own residential centre for people with
health problems.*

Appendix 2
Useful publications

See Appendix 1 for addresses of organizations mentioned here, and the list at the end of this book of other useful publications by Class Publishing. Class Publishing will be publishing further books on MS – please contact them for more information at the address given on p. iv.

MS Society publications

MS Matters, the Society's newsletter is published six times a year (and also available on tape cassette), free to members. They also publish many useful booklets and pamphlets such as:

Complementary therapies

Coping and continent

Has your Mum or Dad got MS?

Making the most of life with MS

MS and healthy eating

MS and social security benefits

MS and your home

People with MS in long-term care

Sources of support

Standards of healthcare for people with MS

Treating MS symptoms

Understanding MS research

What is MS?

MS Trust publications

Open Door, the MS Trust's free newsletter for people affected by MS, is published quarterly and several useful booklets are also available free:

MS: What does it mean for me?

My Dad's got MS

Tips for living with MS

Other publications

Alternative Medicine and Multiple Sclerosis, by A.C. Bowling, published by Demos Publishing, 2001 (associated website: www.ms-cam.org) ISBN 1 888 799528

BT Guide for Disabled People (available free from any BT shop by dialling Freefone 0800 800150 [voice] or 0800 243123 [text]. The guide can also be supplied in large print, braille or audiocassette tape)

Caring at Home, by Nancy Koher, published by National Extension College, 18 Brooklands Avenue, Cambridge CB2 2HN (Tel: 01223 400200)

The Charities Digest, by Claudia Rios, published by Waterlows Charity & Social Services Publications, updated regularly ISBN 1 857 838033

Choosing a Care Home, published by
Department of Health (available
from your local Health Authority)

Complete MS Body Manual,
by Susie Cornell, available from
PO Box 1270, Chelmsford,
CM2 6BQ, 1996

*Comprehensive Nursing Care in Multiple
Sclerosis*, by June Halper
& Nancy Holland, published by
Medical Publishing, 1997
ISBN 1888799056

*Coping with Dementia: handbook for
carers*, by Health Education Board
Scotland, published by Woodburn
House, Canaan Lane, Edinburgh
EH10 4SG

Coping with Multiple Sclerosis, by
Cynthia Benz, published by
Vermilion, 1996
ISBN 0091813611

Directory for Disabled People, by Ann
Darnbrough & Derek Kinrade,
published by Wendy Botwright,
Prentice Hall, Campus 400,
Maylands Avenue,
Hemel Hempstead HP2 7EZ,
Tel: 01442 882058

Disability Rights Handbook, by Judith
Patterson, published by Disability
Alliance Educational and Research
Association, London
(Contact 020 7247 8759
for ordering details)

*Disabled Access Guide to London's West
End Theatres*, 4th edn, published
regularly by Artsline, London
(The disabled access guide to 52
theatres in London's West End,

produced under the Society of
London Theatre's Disabled
Audiences Project with funding
from the Arts Council of England's
New Audiences Programme. Order
from website www.artsline.org.uk)

Door to Door, by Department of
Transport, availabe free of charge
from the Mobility Advice and
Vehicle Information Service
(MAVIS)

*Eating and MS – information and
recipes*, by Susan Fildes, published
by MS Resource Centre, 1994
(Contact them directly on
01206 505 444)

Emotional Reactions to MS, by Julia
Segal, published by the MS
Resource Centre, 1994 (Contact
them directly on 01206 505 444)

*Employment: guidance and code of
practice*. Stationery Office, London
(Order directly on 0870 600 5522)

*A Garden For You: a practical guide to
tools, equipment and design for older
people and people with disabilities*,
by Fred Walden, published by the
Disabled Living Foundation, 1997
ISBN 0 901 90869X

*Gardens of England and Wales: open for
charity 2003*, published annually
by The National Gardens Scheme
ISBN 0 900 558369

*Grow It Yourself: gardening with a
physical disability*, by Roddy
Llewellyn, Ann Davies OBE,
published by Hutchinson Children's
Books, 1993

A Guide to Grants for Individuals in Need, published by the Directory of Social Change, Liverpool/London, 2002 (updated regularly)
ISBN 1 903 991242

Health and Advice for the Traveller, by Department of Health, published by DoH (available from Post Offices or DoH)

Historic House and Gardens, Castles and Heritage Sites. Published by Hunter Publishing 2001
ISBN 0 953 142671

Holiday Care Guide to Accessible Travel, published by the Holiday Care Service (Contact them directly at HCS, 2nd Floor, Imperial Buildings, Victoria Road, Horley, Surrey, RH6 7PZ. Tel: 01293 774535)

How to Get Equipment for Disability, by Michael Mandelstam, published by Jessica Kinglsey Publishers, 116 Pentonville Road, London N1 9JB, Tel: 020 7833 2307
ISBN 1853021903

However Will You Cope? by Michael Wates (discusses experiences of disabled mothers), published by National Childbirth Trust, 1996 (Contact NCT directly on 08709 908040 to order)

McAlpine's Multiple Sclerosis, by WB Matthews (ed), published by Churchill Livingston, 1998
ISBN 0 443 050082 (an expensive book for specialists)

Me and My Shadow, by Carole Mackie & Sue Brattle, published by Aurum Press, 1999
ISBN 1 845 106279

Multiple Sclerosis – the 'at your fingertips' guide, by Professor Ian Robinson, Dr Stuart Neilson and Dr Frank Clifford Rose, published by Class Publishing, 2002
ISBN 1 872362 94 X

Multiple Sclerosis: the guide to treatment and management, 5th edn, by William A. Sibley, published by Demos Publishing, 2001
ISBN 1 888 799544
(Previous editions were under the title *Therapeutic Claims in Multiple Sclerosis*. This book is also available at www.msif.org and from the MSIF – see Appendix for address.)

Multiple Sclerosis – a personal exploration, by A. Burnfield, published by Souvenir Press, 1996
ISBN 0 285 650181

MS, Pregnancy and Parenthood, by Judy Graham, published by MS Resource Centre, 1996 (contact directly on 01206 505444)

Multiple Sclerosis – the natural way, by Richard Thomas, published by Viga Books, 2002
ISBN 1843330369

The National Trust Handbook 2003, published annually by The National Trust 2003
ISBN 0 707 80342 X

Open Door, published by Artsline,
London (A disabled access guide to
fringe theatres in London. The first
edition has been researched by
Artslines' team of access workers,
who are all disabled people
themselves. Order from website
www.artsline.org.uk)

*Places That Care: the guide to places of
interest with access for the elderly and
disabled*, by Michael Yarrow,
published by Grub Street, 1999

Standing in the Sunshine, by Cari Loder,
published by Century, 1996,
ISBN 0712676392

*Taking Time for Me: how caregivers can
deal effectively with stress*,
by K.L. Karr, published by
Prometheus Books, 1993
ISBN 0879757795

Therapeutic Claims in Multiple Sclerosis,
see *Multiple Sclerosis: the guide to
treatment and management*

Traveller's Guide to Health, by the
Department of Health, London
(Contact DoH for a copy)

*What to Look For in a Private or
Voluntary Registered Home*
(Factsheet No 17), published by
Counsel and Care

With a Little Help, published by the
Disabled Living Foundation

Publications by RADAR
Copies of the following factsheets are
available from RADAR. Telephone for
latest prices on 020 7250 3222.

*Assessment centres and driving
instruction*

*Car control manufacturers, suppliers and
fitters*

Cash help for mobility needs

*Discounts and concessions available to
disabled people on the purchase of cars
and other related items*

Driving licences

*Exemption from vehicle excise duty
(VED)*

Insurance

*Meeting the cost of adaptations –
Housing Fact Sheet 2*

Motoring accessories

Motoring with a wheelchair

Relief from VAT and car tax

Index

PRIORITY ORDER FORM

Cut out or photocopy this form and send it (post free in the UK) to:

Class Publishing Priority Service   Tel: **01752 202 301**
FREEPOST (PAM 6219)
Plymouth PL6 7ZZ   Fax: **01752 202 333**

Please send me urgently   *Post included*
(tick boxes below)   *price per copy (UK only)*

☐ **Managing your Multiple Sclerosis**   £17.99
Practical advice to help you manage your multiple sclerosis (ISBN 1 85959 071 3)

☐ **Multiple Sclerosis – the 'at your fingertips' guide**   £17.99
(ISBN 1 872362 94 X)

☐ **Sexual Health for Men – the 'at your fingertips' guide**   £17.99
(ISBN 1 85959 011 X)

☐ **Beating Depression – the 'at your fingertips' guide**   £17.99
(ISBN 1 85959 063 2)

☐ **High Blood Pressure – the 'at your fingertips' guide**   £17.99
(ISBN 1872362 81 8)

☐ **Positive Action for Health and Wellbeing**   £17.99
(ISBN 1 85959 040 3)

☐ **Heart Health – the 'at your fingertips' guide**   £17.99
(ISBN 1 85959 009 8)

TOTAL _____

Easy ways to pay

Cheque: I enclose a cheque payable to Class Publishing for £ _____

Credit card: Please debit my

☐ Mastercard   ☐ Visa   ☐ Switch   ☐ Amex

Number _____   Expiry date _____

Name _____

My address for delivery is _____

_____

Town _____ County _____ Postcode _____

Telephone number *(in case of query)* _____

Credit card billing address if different from above _____

_____

Town _____ County _____ Postcode _____

Class Publishing's guarantee: remember that if, for any reason, you are not satisfied with these books, we will refund all your money, without any questions asked. Prices and VAT rates may be altered for reasons beyond our control.

Have you found **Managing your Multiple Sclerosis: Practical in-depth information to help you manage your multiple sclerosis** useful and practical? If so, you may be interested in other books from Class Publishing.

Multiple Sclerosis – the 'at your fingertips' guide £14.99
Professor Ian Robinson, Dr Stuart Neilson and Dr Frank Clifford Rose

Straightforward and positive answers to all your questions about MS, with over 200 real questions included from people with MS and their families. Armed with this book, you will feel able to cope with the challenges that MS presents and live a full and active life.

'An invaluable resource.'
Jan Hatch, MS Society

Beating Depression – the 'at your fingertips' guide £14.99
Dr Stefan Cembrowicz and Dr Dorcas Kingham

Depression is one of the most common illnesses in the world – affecting up to one in five people at some time in their lives. *Beating Depression* shows sufferers and their families that they are not alone. Written by two medical experts, it offers tried and tested techniques for overcoming depression.

'A sympathetic and understanding guide.'
Marjorie Wallace, Chief Executive, SANE

Positive Action for Health and Wellbeing
Dr Brian Roet £14.99

Dr Roet explains simply and clearly about the positive steps you can take to promote your own health and wellbeing.

'Over the years I have read countless self-help books and none helped. No other book has ever had this effect on me.'
S. G., Hampshire

Sexual Health for Men – the 'at your fingertips' guide
NEW TITLE £14.99
Dr Philip Kell and Vanessa Griffiths

This practical handbook answers hundreds of real questions from men with sexual problems and their partners. Up to 50% of men in the UK aged over 60 have major problems with sexual dysfunction – though they need not have, if they take appropriate action.

High Blood Pressure – the 'at your fingertips' guide £14.99
Dr Julian Tudor Hart, Dr Tom Fahey with Professor Wendy Savage

The authors use all their years of experience as blood pressure experts to answer your questions on high blood pressure, and the more you understand about your high blood pressure – the easier it is to bring it down – and keep it down.

'Readable and comprehensive information.'
*Dr Sylvia McLaughlan, Director General,
The Stroke Association*

Heart Health – the 'at your fingertips' guide
Dr Graham Jackson £14.99

This practical handbook, written by a leading cardiologist, answers all your questions about heart conditions and tells you how to keep your heart healthy, or – if it has been affected by heart disease in some way – how to make it as strong as possible.

'Contains the answers the doctor wishes he had given if only he'd had the time.'
Dr Thomas Stuttaford, The Times